CoDiscovery

*Exploring the Legacy of
Robert F. Barkley, D.D.S.*

Paul A. Henny, D.D.S.

CoDiscovery

Exploring the Life and Legacy of Robert F. Barkley, D.D.S.

Copyright ©2025 Co-Discovery Press, 3rd Edition

ISBN Hard Cover: 9798988896005

ISBN Soft Cover: 9798988896012

ISBN E-Book: 9798988896029

CoDiscovery

*Exploring the Legacy of
Robert F. Barkley, D.D.S.*

Table of Contents

Foreword

My journey in dentistry began in Natal, Brazil, in the late 1990s. The golden era of dentistry was over due to a government initiative to correct an imbalance in the national distribution of dentists. The outcome: a four-fold increase in the number of clinicians, no improvement in distribution, a dramatic increase in dentists practicing in metropolitan areas, intense intra-professional competition, lower fees, and a decrease in the quality of care. Many dentists subsequently left the profession soon after graduation and transitioned into more promising careers. My development took a turn for the better after stopping by the dental school library in search of something to read. Little did I know that what I found that day would dramatically change the arc of my career; it was titled: *"A Philosophy of the Practice of Dentistry"* by L.D. Pankey and William J. Davis.

After graduation, I was eager to put my training to good use, earn a decent living, and help my patients in significant ways, but many of my patients were much less enthusiastic. As time passed and the number of new patients increased, the complexity of their problems increased as well. Because we didn't want to refer out too many patients, we dedicated ourselves to elevating our skills: I pursued postgraduate work in prosthodontics and implant dentistry, while my wife Marcela, specialized in endodontics.

Simultaneously, I searched for ways to improve my case acceptance rate by referencing Dr. Pankey's book, a habit that became my psychological refuge. The different way of practicing described in the book appealed to me on a very deep level, but I struggled to understand the entire meaning of "Know your Work, Know your Patients, Know Yourself and Apply your Knowledge."

Ten years passed as we worked on better ways to know our work and apply our knowledge. I traveled to the United States to attend a year-long implant residency at UAB (and later, specialty training in prosthodontics), where I found another paradigm-shifting book titled *The Exceptional Dental Practice: Why Good Enough Isn't Good Enough,* by William Lockard Jr., DDS. Upon returning to Brazil, we combined our comprehensive care philosophy with more extensive new patient interviews. My developmental journey caused me to repeatedly run across the name Bob Barkley, and the words *Codiscovery* and *CoDiagnosis.* After reading many articles on Lynn Carlisle's *In a Spirit of Caring* website, we started to integrate Bob's teaching philosophy and everything took a turn for the better. Many patients who previously struggled to make good decisions, started to draw their own values-driven conclusions and ask me to help them create more optimal health futures!

This book will help you learn the principles and strategies inside every successful relationship-based, health-centered practice. However, I must warn you that success requires a significant amount of personal work, as you'll have to clarify who you are, create an optimized vision of your preferred future, understand who you want to become, who you want to serve, and what you'll need to do to make it all happen.

I first learned about Paul Henny after reading his *Bob Barkley Study Club* Facebook posts, and because of those communications, I flew to the United States to attend a BBSC meeting in Scottsdale, Arizona. There I met Jon Barkley (Bob's son), Paul, Gary DeWood, Gary Takacs, Mary Osborne, Brian Vence, Alan Stern, Mac McDonald, Matt Standridge, Johnson Hagood, Kevin Dougherty, and Jeff Baggett. I then went on to attend more workshops and met Charley Varipapa, Michelle Lee, Alice Lam, Rodney Baier, and many others. I also traveled to Macomb, IL, with Paul and Jon to see where his father lived and practiced. Along the way, I saw where Bob grew up, attended school, practiced, his homes, the plane crash site, and his final resting place. The timing of this book couldn't be better as American dentists face challenges similar to what occurred in Brazil over twenty years ago. By reading this book, you will have a better understanding of the past, the present, and the exciting future that personalized, health-centered dentistry can bring into your life.

Frederico Diego Lima, DDS

Introduction

Other countries offer prime examples of how everyone can lose when society's demands dilute a profession toward mediocrity...Only a new health-centered philosophy of dentistry at all levels of society can avert a collision with mediocrity worldwide. Furthermore, the traditional approach is difficult to insure without promoting mediocre care...[1]

So begins the introduction to Bob Barkley's landmark book, Successful Preventive Dental Practices. In it, Bob said that the only way to avoid a profession-wide state of mediocrity was to nurture within each person their "latent sense of responsibility so they may become independently healthy."

To Bob, independent health represented the first step toward success because independent health can move a person away from a state of long-term decline toward more stable and optimal functioning. Independent health creates an opportunity for a behaviorally astute care team to shift a person's attention toward a preferred future through a process of planned excellence. Bob also knew that facilitating a mental shift, "getting people to think inductively," required dentists to develop "a renewal of purpose," that's only possible through the development of a different mindset.

Bob was well ahead of his time. As an apostate of the "drill, fill, and bill" culture (put on steroids by insurance company payment patterns), he was dentistry's biggest disruptor. Bob fought against the insanity by focusing his attention on global solutions ranging from dental school curriculum changes to the many challenges associated with running a private practice. Additionally, Bob was changed by his journey: "As my philosophy of dental care matured, my self-image slowly changed from that of a "healer" to one of an interested, empathetic teacher of health who is also capable of providing good restorative dentistry."[2]

The purpose of this book is to help you find your own pathway. The beginning point relates to your role in your patients' lives, something that must be clarified and refined. That process will stretch, challenge, and occasionally push you outside of your comfort zone. However, you'll become wiser as a result—you'll learn *when* and *when not* to apply your knowledge.

To make all of the key information accessible, I have included the relevant thinking of L.D. Pankey, Nate Kohn, Jr., Carl Rogers, Carl Jung, Avrom King, Ben Singer, Wilson Southam, Charles Sorensen, Harold Wirth, Rich Green, Mike Schuster, Bill Strupp, and others who were major influencers on Bob and/or vice versa. That's important because we need to appreciate the shoulders we stand upon.

Additionally, I have included a detailed discussion of Bob Barkley's Three Phase Adult Education, combined with various perspectives, concepts, and anecdotes. Despite the extensive amount of history, I wrote this book to inspire the future — your future, as the final story will be written by you. You have to decide how to best fit all of the pieces together, as well as figure out how to live them out in your life.

~ Paul A. Henny, D.D.S., December 4, 2025

In Appreciation

To my wife, Betsy, for her love, support, and encouragement during the long creation process.

To my children Julianne, Evan, and Allison, and grandchildren Banks and Blaire, for all of their love and understanding.

To Debbie Harden, who invested an incalculable number of hours encouraging, editing, and shepherding this book to its final form.

To Charley Varipapa and Johnson Hagood for their steadfast friendship, support, and collaboration over the past 25 years.

To Stan Kingma, Bob Sweezy, Jon Barkley, Richard Green, Gary Takacs, Brian Vence, Mike Schuster, Walter Doyle, Bill Lockard, Jr., Mac McDonald, Jeff Baggett, Frederico Lima, Joan Forrest, Frank Graziano, Dennis Stiles, Robert Spreen, Gary DeWood, Mary Osborne, Michelle Lee, Alice Lam, Kevin Kwiecien, Alan Stern, Kevin Dougherty, and Bill Strupp for believing in the value of my work and for their unwavering support.

To my exceptional Care Team, who helped me develop, implement, and refine these concepts.

To all of my friends associated with The Bob Barkley Study Club, The Pankey Institute, The Dawson Academy, and the American Equilibration Society.

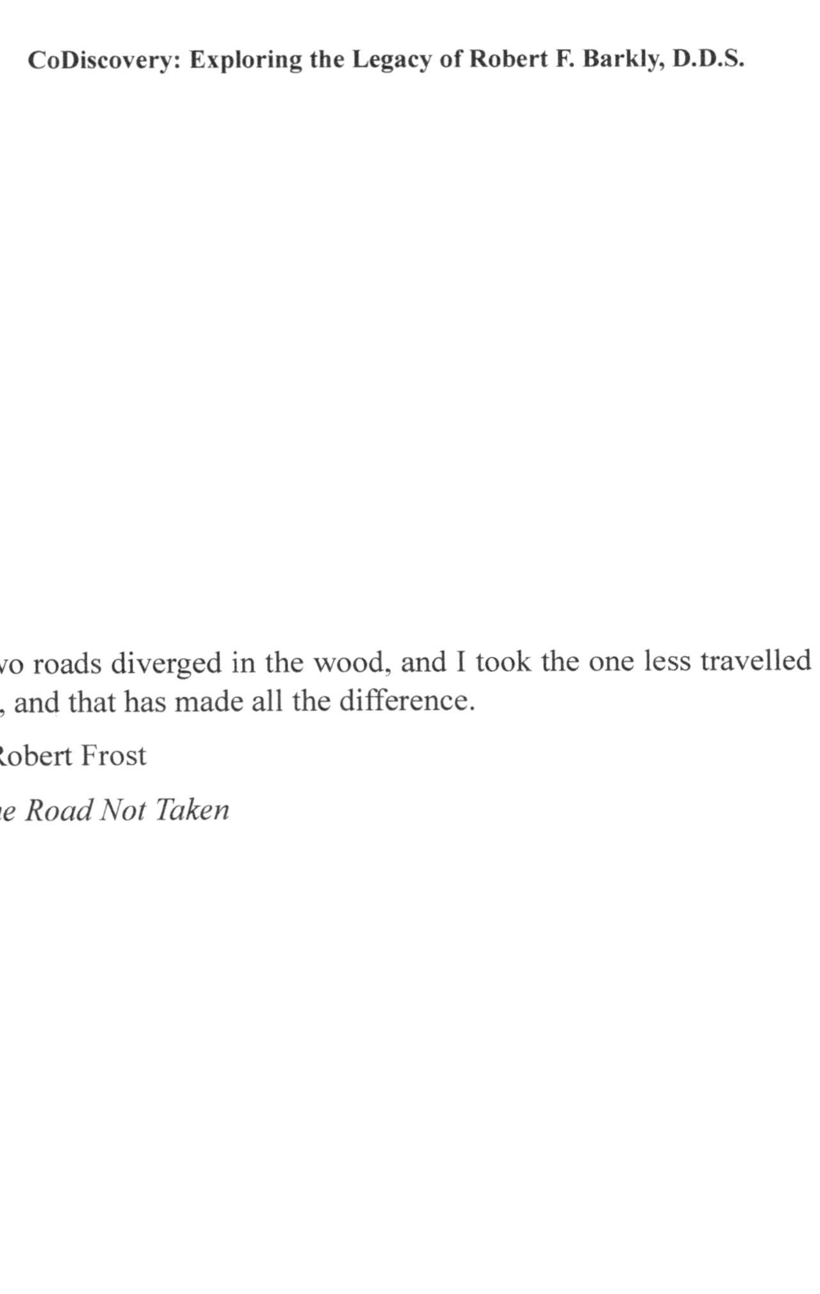

Two roads diverged in the wood, and I took the one less travelled by, and that has made all the difference.

~Robert Frost

The Road Not Taken

Chapter 1
The Origin Of Behavioral Dentistry

Behavioral Dentistry was pioneered by L.D. Pankey after meeting Carl Jung, studying with George Crane, PhD, and reading hundreds of books on psychology, personality, and human motivation.[3] Bob Barkley, a student of Dr. Pankey, took what he had learned from Dr. Pankey to the next level by working closely with Nate Kohn, Jr, PhD, an educational psychologist. Nate was an ideal sounding board as Bob struggled to implement his knowledge. Much of the struggle was related to the dramatically different demographics of Macomb, IL, compared to Coral Gables, Florida. Unlike Coral Gables, the average person in McDonough County farmed, worked in a farming-related business, ran a small business supporting the community, or worked at Western Illinois University.[4] Consequently, most people couldn't afford what they needed on a comprehensive level, so they let their dental problems go until they were intolerable, and made short-term, relief-oriented decisions that undermined their long-term health.

Since Bob grew up in nearby Ipava, he was faced with a conundrum he described as "forced to practice dentistry for the masses or the classes."[5] He was acutely aware that practicing dentistry primarily "for the classes" was financially limiting, so he decided to pursue the development of his low-appreciation-for-fine-dentistry patients instead. Bob's new mission: to help more patients value health-centered dentistry, as doing so saved them money *and* improved their health and appearance. That was an ambitious goal, as only a small percentage of the Macomb area citizens viewed dentistry as a health-centered profession.

Nate Kohn helped Bob create his own expression of the Cross of Dentistry.[6]

1. By getting to know himself better

2. By getting to know his patients in deeper, more meaningful ways
3. By further advancing his clinical skills
4. By applying his knowledge in a more sophisticated and psychologically sound fashion

Nate said that most people have a hidden desire to take better care of themselves that isn't verbalized due to past experiences, distorted memories, financial pressure, or other social influences. He challenged Bob to create a process of self-discovery that would allow each person to explore the value of maintaining a fully functional, attractive dentition over their lifetime. Nate told Bob that if he could figure out how to do that, he would discover most people would choose health and restoration over extractions and dentures. Together, they developed *Three Phase Adult Education*, the engine that would drive Bob's preventive-restorative practice for ten years.

There are countless situations, and restorative dentistry is one of them, in which an overemphasis on speed destroys efficiency. A sound practice depends on our ability to respect and relate to each patient as an individual. That can't be done unless we learn to recognize the differences that make each person unique and are able to slow ourselves down to the tempo of each of our other patients.

~Loren Miller, D.D.S.,

Founding Co-Director of The Pankey Institute

New Opportunities in Dental Practice (1980)

Chapter 2
Who Was Bob Barkley?

Robert F. Barkley was born 225 miles southwest of Chicago in Table Grove, Illinois on August 23, 1930. He was raised with his two sisters, Louise and Carolyn, during the Great Depression. Bob's father was a coal miner, and mother—a schoolteacher. In 1937, his family rented a small farm near Ipava, 24 miles east of Macomb. There, Bob attended V.I.T. High School, a consolidated school where he played football, basketball, baseball, and bass violin.[7]

After graduation, Bob attended Western Illinois University in Macomb, where he studied a pre-dental curriculum while playing in the WIU orchestra. He was accepted into Northwestern University School of Dentistry in the fall of 1951 and began his studies there in the summer of 1952. Bill Lockard, Jr., who would become a visiting faculty member of The Pankey Institute, was his classmate.

Bob assumed multiple part-time jobs to help manage his tuition costs, including being a taxi driver, working at a local hospital, and working in used car sales. Along the way, he burned the proverbial candle at both ends to the degree that the photographer taking his graduation photograph commented, "Young man, I don't know what you are doing, but I see and study a lot of faces every day, and you had better slow down, or change your lifestyle if you want to live a long a productive life."[8] But Bob was an avid learner and had no intention of slowing down after graduating on an accelerated track. He would go on to become a pillar of his community, husband, father to Kevin, David, Jon, Sara, and Ann, an Air Force Dental Officer, an airplane pilot, contributor to multiple professional journals, author of the legendary *Successful Preventive Dental Practices*, owner and operator of a practice consultancy, curriculum and admissions advisor to multiple dental schools, and member of The Pankey Institute Planning Committee and Board of Trustees. Additionally, Bob became the most popular speaker in the history of dentistry (often speaking 8-9 times a month around the country up until the time of his death).

After completion of his two-year commitment to the Air Force, Bob set up a scratch practice in downtown Macomb in a second-floor space that overlooked the courthouse square, which was within walking distance of his growing family; the year was 1957. Bob described Macomb as "the largest town between Ipava and the Mississippi River."[9] Most county residents were middle class or lower, and the average 60-year-old wore a partial or full denture. Bob quickly outgrew the downtown location and moved into a free-standing building near the community hospital.

Like most recent graduates, Bob believed he was practicing a superior brand of dentistry; however, within a relatively short period of time, he noticed that a significant amount of his work was failing. His conclusion: there must be a problem with his technique and the quality of materials. Consequently, Bob learned more about cast gold restorations. "I assured myself that better quality repairs were the answer," he said.

While the changes in techniques and materials increased Bob's net income, they generated an unanticipated side effect—some people left his practice. Additionally, he developed a reputation for being a "gold man,"[10] a laudable descriptor within dental circles that most Macomb citizens viewed in a more negative light. To many, Bob had gone "big time" and left them behind by failing to address their highest priority—minimizing expenses.

In 1960, Bob attended Dr. Clyde Schuyler's lecture and shared his small-town struggles. Dr. Schuyler told him that he needed to offer a broader range of clinical services (what Bob would later refer to as "decathlon dentistry") because he felt that Bob "could sell more things than he knew how to do."[11] Dr. Schuyler's words motivated Bob to pursue comprehensive restorative training under L.D. Pankey.

Bob's new skills allowed him to develop more sophisticated treatment plans with higher case fees. In Bob's mind, the new strategy would lead to more success on all levels, as the superiority of his planning and skill set were obvious—to him. Unfortunately, many of his patients didn't see it that way: "Are there really that many problems in my mouth? And if so, why can't you just fix them right now?" Bob soon realized that he had reached another philosophical crossroads: Should he practice dentistry the best way he knew, or should he practice dentistry the way his patients wanted, and accept all of the associated frustrations and failures as being a necessary part of small-town dentistry? "It seemed that a decision had to be made whether to work for the classes or the masses. Reluctantly, I chose the former. I decided that I would offer what I knew was best for the patient and let the chips fall where they may."[12] And fall they did, as more and more patients left the practice; some left disgruntled, while others left confused—and as a sensitive, empathic person, it broke his heart. Yet, the worst was yet to come.

During that time, a former V.I.T. classmate (one of his favorite cheerleaders) came in seeking help. She told Bob that she was unable to smile in public as her fourth child had "drawn out all of the calcium" from her teeth and that she wanted dentures. Bob approached the situation with caution, as he was fully aware of past failures to sell proper restorative dentistry under similar circumstances. So, Bob tried a different strategy that day. He showed her how she could improve her hygiene skills, and then proposed a Phase I Plan that could be revisited when her finances improved. The plan was agreed to and an appointment to begin was set. But when the day arrived, she didn't show up. Later, Bob discovered why when he saw her in public struggling to wear immediate dentures. She *"committed dental suicide"* in another office.[13]

The experience was so traumatic that it catalyzed a shift in how Bob perceived the practice of dentistry. It also set the stage for many creative solutions he would later share. Bob wanted "to make prevention pay off," ensuring—especially when the person couldn't afford extensive restorative dentistry—*the deployment of an initial preventative strategy would stop disease progression and allow the person more time to prepare themselves financially for proper restoration.* Toward that end-goal, Bob studied biological and behavioral dentistry: From Drs. C.C. Bass and Sumter Arnim, he learned more about the management of dental caries and periodontal disease from Paul Keys, DDS, MS. He learned how to use a phase contrast microscope. Additionally, Nathan Kohn, Jr., PhD, taught Bob about strategic interpersonal communication, the emotional and psychological requirements necessary to achieve behavior change, as well as how to facilitate optimal learning.[14]

Bob Barkley's most recognized legacy is associated with his barnstorming of a preventive dentistry program that leveraged experiential learning. The five-day program was based on the number of days it takes a person to be able to observe cessation of bleeding after they've elevated their oral hygiene skills. Bob's Disease Control Program,"[15] began with the use of a phase contrast microscope, which helped each person learn that dental plaque = microbiome. The interactive learning process was:

- Personalized (and targeted only at patients who demonstrated active disease)
- Relevant
- Goal-oriented
- Well-coached
- Supported new habit formation
- Facilitated positive change

Each patient learned how to stop bacterial and spirochete destruction as well as the long-term implications of not doing so. For those efforts, Bob became known as the "Pied Piper of Plaque" and the "Billy Graham of Dentistry."[16] Despite the program's effectiveness, the insurance industry refused to compensate dentists for the time and resources committed to providing it. As a result, Bob lamented that true preventive, health-centered dentistry wasn't likely to get much of a foothold if dental insurance companies refused to support it.

In *Successful Preventive Dental Practices*, Bob shared a conversation he had with the dentist-executive of a non-profit dental service corporation, who told Bob that compensating dentists for their time and resources used to teach their patients about prevention "was an open invitation to fraud" as there wasn't any way to prove they had done it. Bob said, "It would be intriguing to know how your company currently determines whether or not a prophylaxis or other traditional preventive measure has been carried out…"[17]

The bottom line: dental service corporations and private insurance companies possessed an inherent distrust of dentists, and subsequently, they didn't believe dentists were likely to do the right things for their patients without direct supervision. As a result, the relationship between dentists and insurance companies remained adversarial and bound to a *remedial philosophy:* What has gone wrong since your last visit? Is there anything we need to fix or repair?—instead of evolving into a more health-centered philosophy that promotes self-ownership, goal formation, collaboration, and health by *asking questions* such as: What would you like to see happen over time? How can I help you achieve your goals?

Bob would go on to create a three-part patient development method that was designed to promote in each person:

- Better understanding of their situation (by elevating their awareness and facilitating the creation of relevance)
- Better understanding of the long-term implications associated with various decisions (values clarification and reorganization)
- Ownership of their problems (boundary development),
- Participation

As you can see, Bob Barkley's influence was broad, deep, and impressive. His untimely death in a chartered plane crash on August 13, 1977, brought a tragic end to a meteoric career that was rapidly reshaping the profession of dentistry.

Bob's influence lives on through those who heard him speak, read his book, saw his instructional videos, and leveraged his knowledge to create genuine, collaborative, health-centered practices. The progressive nature of Bob's thinking and techniques remain more important today than ever, as most of our profession remains mired in a remedial, repair-centric philosophy that's driven by insurance company payment patterns.

Chapter 3
What Is "Person-Centered" Dentistry?

Some of the terminology in this book has the potential to create confusion, so let me define a few commonly used phrases before we advance further into the text: The terms *health-centered, person-centered, personalized, humanistic,* and *helping,* mean similar things to most people who practice this style of dentistry. Each term implies that we're limited with regard to *how much* health we can create or maintain in another person. It's generally agreed that we can help others in moments of crisis, and we can certainly make many situations better, but health isn't static, and it usually cannot remain stable without some level of participation by a person who has decided to take ownership of their situation.

The key takeaway here is that **health represents a *personal* pursuit, and therefore, it's personally defined**. In other words, *optimal health* represents something different to each person. On that point, Bob Barkley said, "The real measure of health is not the utopian absence of all disease; rather, health represents the ability of a person to function effectively within their given environment."[18]

A person cannot remain healthy unless they are making health-centered decisions in the areas of diet, exercise, mindfulness, choosing pro-social behavior, and so forth. Additionally, a dentist can be utilized by a health-conscious person to advance their health. Still, if the chosen dentist isn't philosophically health-centered, then the person's goals may never be achieved.

If a patient isn't behaving in a health-centered fashion relative to dentistry, it's likely due to one of four reasons:

1. They have never experienced a health-centered relationship with a dentist in the past and therefore do not know how to collaborate.

2. In the past, they have tried to collaborate with a dentist in a health-centered fashion, but it only led to more failures and frustrations, and they subsequently became cynical about what the dental profession could do for them.

3. They are health-centered at heart, but they are experiencing financial limitations that force them to remain in a basic care/remedial mode.

4. They don't value dental health and choose to use dental services only for emergency situations.

A *health-centered* or *person-centered* practice can help in all of these people, but tends to focus its time, energy, and resources on assisting the top three types of patients through clearly sharing their philosophy via a health-centered leadership, and by establishing a trust*worthy* relationship within which the person can navigate, collaborate, set goals, and involve themselves in the process.

Wilson Southam was a major investor in *The Cox Group*®—a Canadian dental equipment manufacturer located in Stoney Creek, Ontario, and was the developer of the first ergonomic dental equipment known as "the dentist's cockpit." Wilson was an avid supporter of health-centered dentistry, and because he was also a newspaper publisher and a film producer, he was very keen on the meaning of words. Wilson felt the term *health-centered* failed to capture the full intention of an ideal practice, so he borrowed the term *person-centered* from Carl Rogers, PhD. Person-centered therapy is somewhat non-directive, in the sense that it's intended to help each person develop their own treatment goals as well as determine the pace at which they'd like to pursue them. On this topic, Wilson said:

The term health-centered was used by Bob Barkley, but I feel that calling it "person-centered" is more appropriate, as it's hard not to have an agenda when health-centeredness is your stated and steadfast goal. So, in my view, we want to be as agenda-free as possible in the beginning of every new relationship so that we can both see if we have enough common ground to successfully work together. In my mind, thinking of ourselves as being person-centered forces us to always be attuned to each person's value system, priorities, experiences, universe, etc., and then help them create their own personalized definition of health. If what they want to do isn't compatible with what we do, then so be it, we can both respectfully exit the relationship without being judgmental.[19] Wilson Southam called his deferential philosophy a *volitional practice*. He believed that truly helping relationships are founded on shared values, priorities, and a clearly defined preferred future. If a relationship required manipulation (emotional, financial, or otherwise) to be maintained, then it was by definition not health-centered.

In an interview with Lynn Carlisle, Wilson said that the unstated thesis of a volitional practice is:

In a health setting of authentic caring and freedom, most people will move toward higher levels of self-care of their own volition. Thus, volitional practice utterly respects the right of individuals to choose what is best for their own health future, and its ultimate objective is to help people help themselves.[20]

Chapter 4
What Are Values And Why Do They Matter?

Values are beliefs that compete as they are proven right, wrong, weak, or strong. Our strongest values, our *primary* values, guide most of our decision-making process. Thus, it's important to understand our primary values and prioritize them in ways that support advancement.

Values are also time-dependent, much like life itself, which comes in the form of seasons. During each season, different values take precedence as priorities, abilities, and resources shift. Primary values are uniquely important to each person and therefore influence behavior in unique ways. Thus, it's impossible to fully understand a person's behavior and decision-making process without first understanding the person on the values level. When we do that, we begin to see the world as they perceive it, hence we begin to understand *why* this issue is more important to them than that issue. From there, we are able to play more of an advisory role as the person merges new information into their lattice of values and priorities. Better yet, we can help them see that their oral health is an integral part of their total health.

Bob Barkley said:

Values clarification encourages a learner to identify and develop their values and beliefs and it's a process that's based upon trust that the learner is capable of wisely choosing sound concepts following this kind of facilitation. The future of dentistry will be led by those who have clarified their values, are focused on achieving their preferred future, and have developed a humanistic management style that allows them to help others clarify their values and priorities as well. By so doing, both dentists and their patients will become more effective and successful human beings.[21]

The human being cannot live in a condition of emptiness for very long: If he is not growing toward something, he does not merely stagnate; the pent-up potentialities turn into morbidity and despair, and eventually into destructive activities.

~Rollo May

(*Man's Search for Himself,* Souvenir Press, LTD, 1982: p. 27)

Chapter 5
Values Clarification Leads into Vision Formation

If we aspire to create a true relationship-driven practice, we must first help our patients clarify their values and priorities relative to oral health and dentistry as opposed to persuading them, as the act of persuasion risks projection of our values and priorities onto others. Next, we need to facilitate a mental conceptualization of what the person wants the outcome of our collaboration to look and feel like, instead of just allowing them to assume a more passive role in the relationship. That distinction becomes even more important when a person is faced with a complex problem that's expensive and time-consuming to resolve.

Bob Barkley said:

The dentist must help guide the patient's thinking, or in most cases, introspection will not occur. This is true because, without guidance, many dental patients think of dentistry in terms of cost rather than what they would really like for their mouths. In dentistry, such inverted thinking often leads to senseless extractions or inferior repairs.[22]

When we spend the appropriate amount of time facilitating the expression of what a person wants to see happen, the pathway toward achieving it narrows. On this, Avrom King said, "As a person's values become more and more clear, the range of choices narrows until, ultimately, there is no choice, and then one is free!"

A person's primary values represent a cluster of interrelated beliefs that are so fundamental, so *core*, they function as guideposts throughout the decision-making process. Additionally, as a person becomes clearer about what they'd like to see happen on the physical and psychological levels, it becomes easier for them to see what they'll need to do to achieve it.

Our primary values lead to feelings, which then drive our behavior. Therefore, emotion catalyzes enduring change. When a feelings-driven vision is uploaded into the subconscious mind, it changes what a person will pay attention to—as well as what they'll ignore.

If we fail to take our patients through a similar process, they won't experience the feelings necessary to catalyze significant change. On that topic, Bob Barkley said:

Our patients' beliefs are what drive their decisions and behavior. Dentists who learn to avoid explanations in favor of helping patients think more inductively will be the ones who are most successful at positively influencing their patients to make better decisions and to maintain long-term, health-centered behavior.[23]

Chapter 6
Lindsey D. Pankey, D.D.S.

L.D. Pankey graduated in 1924 from the University of Louisville College of Dentistry and immediately purchased a practice in New Castle, Kentucky. He would only stay for 18 months due to a life-changing experience, "…one day after lunch, I went to the post office where I found a letter that would forever change my life." In the letter, his mother shared that she had all her teeth extracted and was wearing dentures, "This has been the unhappiest experience of my life…I hope you are not doing to your patients what has been done to me." She was 42 and lived to the age of 87, "and I don't think she had a happy day the rest of her life. Those dentures completely changed her looks, her self-assurance, and her self-confidence," L.D. said. [24]

That seminal experience caused a philosophical shift in Dr. Pankey's mind as he was, in fact, frequently "doing to his patients what has been done to me." L.D. soon left New Castle to start a new life in Coral Gables, Florida, with an entirely new focus:

I spent the rest of my life trying to learn, use, and teach other dentists to give their patients: (1) Comfort, (2) Function, (3) Health, and (4) Esthetics. This can only be done by saving people's teeth. The shock of it all and the considerable thought I gave it, opened the door to a vision that the dentist's responsibility and goal should be to save people's teeth for a lifetime, if at all possible…Early in my career, I felt the need to extend the holistic concept – to see the patient, practitioner, and the practice of dentistry as balanced and distinct, but interrelated entities.

L.D. Pankey became a student of people *and* dentistry, which led him to travel across the globe to learn, organize, integrate, and teach. He co-developed a dental rehabilitation process known as the *Pankey-Mann-Schuyler (PMS) Technique,* taught at *Oral Rehabilitation Seminars (ORS),*[25] in addition to *A Philosophy of the Practice of Dentistry* lectures. His 3-day courses became so popular that the Dupont Plaza Hotel was selected as a permanent teaching location. (It was during that time that Bob Barkley traveled to Miami to train under Dr. Pankey. By 1974, the teacher and student roles merged when L.D. mentioned Bob's work in his *Philosophy* course manual: *"Dr. Barkley, with his Disease Control Program, makes available to all practicing dentists the tools to help patients reduce the incidence of caries and periodontal disease in their own mouths. Getting mouths healthy before treatment and keeping them that way is a worthy objective in itself, and will significantly increase patient acceptance of complete dental care. Perhaps only one-half to two-thirds of the patients can continue with restorative procedures in the beginning, but almost all of them can accept your best services within one year or so. A combination of dental disease control and a holding program will permit this delay in most cases without unduly damaging the patient's dental welfare. The above brief comments on Dr. Barkley's preventive program do not do justice to entirety of his work."*)

As more and more dentists learned about Dr. Pankey's philosophy and how to best apply it, the idea of creating an institute to teach *The Philosophy* in perpetuity bubbled to the surface. Harold Wirth asked, "How would you like to have an institute named after you? It would become a place where dentists from all over the world could come to learn the technique and philosophy."

A curriculum was developed for dentists to attend three once-a-year seminars focused on *The Philosophy* and its psychological, social, and technical application. The L.D. Pankey Foundation, Inc. was simultaneously formed to guide the organization, with *The Pankey Institute* (the Foundation's teaching arm) led by Drs. John Anderson and Loren Miller, starting with a *trial run class.* [26] Loren Miller and John Anderson then offered visiting teaching positions to the top fifteen continuum graduates. That group became known as "The Original Cadre."[27] Those individuals, in combination with countless others, became the shoulders upon which today's Pankey Institute stands.[28]

A short list of current and former organizers, contributors, administrators, and inspirational leaders include, Henry Tanner, Irwin Becker, Peter Dawson, Rose Quick, Chris Sager, Gary DeWood, Dale Sorenson, Lee Ann Brady, Mac McDonald, Alice Lam, Mary Osborne, Joan Unterschuetz, Mark Kleive, Jeff Baggett, Mike Fling, Mike Schuster, Steve Ratcliff, Mike Crete, Mike Rogers, David Swan, Michelle Lee, Dennis Stiles, Kevin Todd Sander, Kevin Kwiecien, Mark Murphy, DeAnne Blazek, Sheri Kay, Kevin Browne, Allison Watts, Brad Portnoy, Denny Byrne, Mark Collis, Ed Mukamal, Frank Graziano, Ricki Braswell, Barry Polansky, Deborah Bush, Gary Takacs, Glenda Owen, Jay Anderson, James Otten, Jim Kessler, Nancy Ward, Clayton Davis, Eben DeArmond, Jim Kinkaid, Steve Malone, Charlie Ward, Tal Wilkins, Ed Zebovitz, Mark Piper, Herb Blumenthal, Steve Carstensen, DeWitt Wilkerson, Todd Davis, John Droter, Glenn Kidder, Bill Gregg, Jim Fondriest, Susan Hollar, Robert Spreen, Steve Hart, Ozzie Osbjornson, and many others.

The two most important days in your life are the day you were born and the day you find out why.

~Mark Twain

Chapter 7
What Are Philosophy Statements?

The pathway to achieving greater efficiency, integrating new technology, reducing no-shows, and improving case acceptance rates runs through the creation of actionable goals. But before we can make significant progress in these areas, we must create a written *Practice Philosophy Statement.* Why? Because a written Philosophy Statement is our *Practice Constitution* that guides all future decisions.

Our *Philosophy* is based on our clarified values and priorities, while our *Mission* is how we apply those values and priorities in the real world. At its core, a dental practice is a complex combination of physical, psychological, and social systems. A written philosophy statement helps us create congruent, philosophically-inspired systems. Philosophically-inspired systems help people to become more aligned, over time. When a person is well-aligned, they grow and contribute to the refinement of the systems. When a person isn't well-aligned, their response is resistance or disruption. Both can occur on the team and patient levels. Resisters and disruptors need to be identified and either aligned or moved out of the practice, as there is no comfortable middle ground when it comes to philosophy. Our philosophy must be clear, lived, protected, and reinforced; otherwise it's nothing more than wishful thinking on a piece of paper.

If you don't have a written Practice Philosophy Statement, I highly recommend make the creation of one a top priority. Goals are essential, but without a written Practice Philosophy to back them up, there's little chance that they will lead you toward your preferred future.

On this topic, Bob Barkley said:

A clarified philosophy of practice helps us to overcome the difficulty of establishing long-term helping relationships with our patients. If we are not clear about what we believe in, then how can we expect others to follow our lead? Even though such long-term relationships are mandatory for long-term success, few dentists intentionally work to establish them prior to examining patients and commencing treatment, rather they begin relationships with others largely based on assumptions. Oftentimes these assumptions are wrong, and this undermines the quality of the relationship over time. Consequently, a dentist's failure to create high-quality, long-term collaborative relationships with their patients leads to a very static and limiting form of practicing. And then after doing so, many dentists wonder why so many of their patients are failing to respond appropriately. Some dentists will even rationalize that their patients don't care about prevention and proper restoration, but in reality, their patient's behavior is not based on their indifference but rather on a lack of appreciation for the value of truly helping relationships on the part of their dentist, and their dentist's inability to establish them.[29]

Bob Barkley was adamant that Philosophy Statements be no more than a single-page, double-spaced document. He felt that a longer document longer wasn't sufficiently concise, and therefore, needed further clarification. Hence, a Philosophy Statement must to be brief and to the point (you may need the facilitation of a practice coach to create one). Below is part of Bob's Philosophy Statement, dated 1972. Note how he designed the document to be iterative, much like how a constitution can be amended over time as circumstances change:

The Purpose of My Practice

The main purpose of my practice is to help my patients prevent dental disease. Science has proven the preventability; it is only a matter of practical application of our knowledge. I want to deal with my patients as complete persons or, even better, with complete families; for only through altering their life's habits in eating and oral hygiene can we hope to achieve lasting results. Whenever we fail in our preventive efforts, it is our goal to provide the best possible corrective treatment. The best we can offer is a lousy substitute for their original healthy oral tissues. All corrective treatment will be considered a potential periodontal problem and will be planned to allow for the greatest ease of achieving an acceptable level of cleanliness.[30]

Bob then went on to describe what he *would* and *would not* do, such as "Artificial dentures shall not be available from my office except for upper dentures as a part of a complete mouth rehabilitation in which lower teeth are being maintained." Finally, Bob designed his practice philosophy statement to be time sensitive and set it up in a diary format that included various commitments and the dates that the changes were made. Some examples:[31]

Aug. '68: Periodontal surgery abandoned during first six months of treatment. Patient's responsibility for periodontal health will be firmly established as the basis for long-term relationships. Surgery will be limited to areas patient proves unmanageable.

Jan '70: PRIMARY PURPOSE OF PRACTICE

ALTERED. My primary purpose is no longer to teach people to control dental disease. Must first get patient to develop their own personal philosophy of dentistry so that their latent sense of responsibility for their health can be developed.

Consider using this helpful format to create your own Philosophy Statement with your Care Team, and keep it updated as your practice evolves.

Note: Philosophy Statements are intra-office management/leadership tools and shouldn't be read to patients, although posting your philosophy statement on the wall, putting it in a brochure, or on your website *is* appropriate. Discussing your philosophy *is* important *after* you have come to know the patient on a deeper level – particularly at the treatment planning/presentation phase.

Chapter 8
Nate Kohn, Jr., PhD

Bob Barkley frequently credited Nate Kohn, Jr., as having a major influence on his career development. Bob and Nate worked together for eight years up until Nate's passing at age 55 in 1970. Bill Brown, who worked with Nate on his Des Moines, Iowa practice, called him, *"the unsung hero of relationship-based dental practice."[32]* Nate held degrees in law, divinity, forestry, and a PhD in educational psychology. Prior to establishing his dental practice consultancy, Nate was an Assistant Professor of Education and the Registrar at University College at Washington University in St. Louis. Bob started working with Nate in 1962 when Nate helped him select team members via personality testing instruments and structured interviews. Nate went on to facilitate the development of Bob's health-centered practice by teaching him about how people learn through the use of Carl Rogers' person-centered model.

Nate famously said:

When a patient leaves your office able to explain to his friends his relationship with you and how it benefits him, immediately, and in years ahead, you have established a relationship with the patient which is the only sound basis for growth of your practice and the development of your profession...Psychologists have discovered that the inability of dentists to establish this type of relationship with their patients is a major contributing factor to the problem as to why more people don't avail themselves to adequate dental care...(and) because of this attitude of the dentist, the patient fails to have the measure of respect, affection, and attachment to the dentist, which he wants, and his dental health is not maintained at a degree that it should be. This results in the dentist not performing services he desires to perform and the patient not becoming a missionary – in a sense of education for the value of dentistry.[33]

As a result, Bob reorganized his new patient examination process around experiential learning and values clarification. "Instead of elaborate explanations and presentations of what we want, or what we feel confident the patient wants, we make a rather concerted effort to get into the patient's frame of reference to discover what he wants to learn or what he feels is relevant," he said.

The collaboration between Bob and Nate led them to co-publish an article titled *The Dentist-Patient Relationship*. Additionally, Nate co-authored the book *Selection, Hiring, and Training of Dental Auxiliaries*, with Edward Green, DDS, in 1970, right before Nate's untimely death.

Question: Have you considered collaborating with a consultant who understands the challenges associated with the creation of a health-centered dental practice?

Chapter 9
Avrom King's Three Tiers Of Dentistry

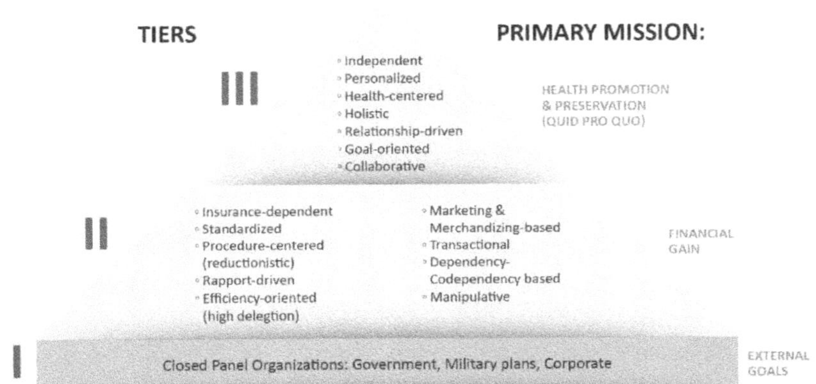

Social psychologist Avrom King was an enthusiastic student of the dental profession, and a close friend of Bob Barkley starting in 1970. Avrom frequently traveled from Phoenix to Macomb to meet with Bob and cross-pollinate on how they could best facilitate an optimal future for the dental profession.[34] Part of that work involved a projection of what Avrom thought the profession would look like in the future based on cultural, professional, and technological meta-trends. Avrom named it the "Three Tiers."[35] Each Tier represented a different business model based upon a different business philosophy and purpose, which then generates different outcomes for dentists and patients under each model:

TIER I: Full third-party funded dentistry wherein treatment is rendered by dentists and other paraprofessionals under pre-paid, capitation, or government funding. Examples: military dentistry, public health clinics, and rent-seeking dental clinics that target government payments as their primary source of income.

Care Type: Reductive, repetitive, remedial, problem-centered, immediate repair-oriented. Treatment is largely "done to" people. "Tooth-centered" as there isn't enough time to develop effective helping relationships with patients on a deeper level or execute long-term strategies, as the patient pool and provider pool are constantly changing.

TIER II: Insurance contract offices, wherein a significant amount of the treatment cost is reimbursed by -and therefore largely mediated by a third-party (non-governmental) payer who has a say-so regarding how much treatment each person is allowed to receive (if they want reimbursement), when they can receive it, and how much providers are compensated for doing the work. Tier II is identifiable by its extensive use of marketing, merchandising, and heuristics (a manipulative approach to communication that triggers decisions most people would not make).

Care Type: Largely reductive, remedial, problem-centered/repair-centered (primarily because insurance plans are structured to function in that fashion). Treatment is largely "done to" people; it is "tooth-centered" because generally speaking, there isn't enough time for dentists and team members to develop deeper, more meaningful, goal-oriented, health-centered relationships with their patients.

TIER III: Private, fee-for-service, relationship-based (developmental), health-centered (collaborative and health-goal oriented), restorative, and regenerative care.

Care Type: Restorative in terms of form, function, and esthetics, or regenerative with regard to guiding or correcting developmental issues such as airway, jaw asymmetries, etc. Treatment is "done with" people; "People-centered." Integrative and holistic, commonly involving collaboration with health-centered (versus disease-centered) physicians and other health care professionals to co-create more optimal outcomes and preferred futures.

The current dental marketplace, is closely following Avrom's projection. Both Tiers I & II are rapidly expanding due to ever-increasing government involvement in combination with consolidation and corporatization. In other words, the majority of the profession is becoming more industrialized with an emphasis on efficiency over relationships, and a concurrent de-emphasis on getting patients more involved.

The generally impersonal Tier I and II business models stand in stark contrast to the Tier III practice model. Health-centered (Tier III) dentistry's expansion into airway management, growth and development, sleep medicine, dietary counseling, etc., has created a tremendous opportunity for those who have prepared themselves to assist—through more effective working relationships—an expanding health-conscious population.

As the broader dental profession devolves into becoming more and more like a highly skilled trade administered by replaceable worker bees and almost entirely controlled by third parties, the highly personalized Tier III patient experience will stand alone as an alternative form of non-industrialized care available to discerning healthcare consumers who have health-centered goals in mind.

Chapter 10
Charles M. Sorensen, MS, PhD

Charles Sorensen met Bob Barkley in 1970, shortly before the unexpected passing of Nate Kohn. Chuck had a PhD in clinical psychology, a PhD in organizational development, and a Master's degree in Theology.[36] Bob and Chuck collaborated on several professional surveys. Bob used to advise dental schools on whom he thought (psychographically speaking) they should enroll. Chuck and Bob later joined forces to create a practice consultancy, which included Dwayne Furman, PhD (a former graduate student of Don Clifton, PhD), and Bud Ham. Eleven practices were under their leadership and development in 1977.

In a 1970 interview in the *Journal of Clinical Orthodontics*, Chuck Sorensen said, "I believe that the mission of a truly health-centered dentist should be to help their patients claim their self-esteem, and not just claim straighter, whiter teeth, or a better bite. They need to help each person to feel better about themselves, help them feel glad to smile, help them to make friends more easily, to get a better job, to be a better lover, parent, and friend."[37]

Chuck believed that the mouth was the most intimate and emotionally sensitive part of the body, and that only "behaviorally sensitive" dentists were capable of successfully operating in that realm for the purpose of helping others "reclaim their self-esteem." Additionally, Chuck believed that other than individuals who were in significant pain or discomfort, most people wouldn't go to see a dentist if they didn't care about how their teeth influenced how they felt about themselves. In other words, most people go to dentists for emotional reasons as well as for objective reasons, yet the emotional reasons are rarely explored or understood.

Chuck also advanced the concept of "missionality"—the desire of a dentist to have a purpose in their life that's significantly greater than the pursuit of fulfilling their own needs. He said that missionality tends to develop in a dentist over time. On that topic, he said:

We have found that a more altruistic sense of mission develops later in some dentists. As they get further into their profession (and they have the potential to grow beyond just being competent with their hands), some discover that they like to help others physically and emotionally. In other words, a stronger sense of mission emerges in some dentists who are able to connect with their patients on deeper, more meaningful levels. [38]

The ability to become more "missional" in dentistry represents a significant shift in perspective. It represents an evolution on the philosophical level that allows a person to enjoy their work in more spiritually profound ways. Chuck said, "Until a dentist discovers a sense of mission, and therefore gains a greater sense of joy and satisfaction from his or her career, they will easily get bored, and progressively lose the personal satisfaction associated with their work as a dentist."[39]

In 1970, Charles Sorensen collaborated on a survey with Bob Barkley and Don Clifton, PhD. Members of the Restorative Academy and the American Academy of Preventive Dentistry were surveyed for the purpose of identifying common characteristics found in "outstanding dentists" as defined by their peer group. Hundreds of dentists were surveyed, including L.D. Pankey and Harold Wirth.[40]

The conclusion of the survey:[41]

The 10 Characteristics of Outstanding Dentists

1. Demonstrate clinical excellence

2. Love working with their hands

3. Are excellence-oriented

4. View dentistry as if it's an art form

5. Conceptualize dentistry as being health-oriented

6. Are personally health-oriented

7. Are behaviorally sensitive

8. Enjoy being around people

9. Enjoy facilitating growth in others

10. Are good at promoting self-responsibility in others

Chuck was convinced that a successful restorative and esthetic dental practice needed to be structured within a *behaviorally sensitive* model. He said:

The simple fact is that people live if they don't have their mouth restored, or have a perfect smile. These people are functionally making a choice between fine dentistry and vacations, boats, furniture, and cars. So, the fine restorative dentist must first become a helper, by helping people to clarify their values, and then, hopefully, help them to place fine comprehensive dentistry higher on their values list.

Question: Is your practice "behaviorally sensitive"? Can you clearly explain your practice's mission and how it plays out each day?

Side Note: Charles Sorensen was recruited by Don Clifton to join his psychographic research company based in Lincoln, Nebraska, initially focused on employee recruitment, strategic hiring, and team development. SRI would later purchase Gallup®, which evolved into *Gallup Learning*, a multimillion-dollar international coaching and leadership development organization. Bob Barkley was interested in influencing how dental schools selected students. He felt that personality characteristics such as communication skills, empathy, missionality, excellence orientation, etc., should be given significant weight in the selection process. Bob wanted to shift the dental profession away from being tooth-centered to person-centered. He felt that dentistry could only become more health-centered if dental schools selected "people-persons" who had an internal drive to help others on a level that was far beyond simply repairing and replacing teeth. Bob used the research findings generated by Charles Sorensen and Don Clifton to work with several dental schools, including the University of Iowa, Loma Linda, USC, and LSU. [42]

A dentist is not just a technician, but a psychologist, social worker, diplomat, educator, and motivator. Like it or not, the product is not dentistry; people must buy our care, skill, and judgment before they place their oral health in our hands.

~ W. J. Davis and L. D. Pankey, *A Philosophy of the Practice of Dentistry*

Chapter 11
The Industrialization Of Dentistry

Despite its restrictions and limitations, Bob Barkley could sense that entrepreneurial dentists viewed the growing availability of dental insurance coverage as a huge business opportunity. By increasing patient volume through the use of delegation, significant profits could be realized in spite of lower compensation levels. Over time, dentists would master the gleaning of insurance plans up to the level of an art form. Avrom King called it *the industrialization of dentistry*, a meta-trend that would eventually destroy the traditional family practice model.

Bob and Avrom were correct, but what they couldn't foresee was the additional impact inflation would have on the profession. The US dollar was taken off the gold standard in 1971,[43] which allowed the US Treasury Department to print currency more freely and the Federal Reserve to game the financial system while attempting to manipulate the economy. That decision influenced dentistry when insurance companies refused to compensate dentists for the inflationary pressure on their practices. Instead, they chose to blame-shift the overhead increases onto dentists by implying that any time a dentist raised his or her fees, they were acting in an "unreasonable" and "uncustomary" fashion. In other words, instead of insurance companies increasing premiums and pay-outs, they manipulated dentists into ignoring their overhead increases due to fear that the insurance companies would drive patients away from their practices. That had the net effect of dental insurance taking on the form of a rapidly devaluing currency. It now takes $7.87 to purchase what $1.00 used to purchase in 1970, yet insurance company yearly maximum allowable amounts have hardly changed during that same period of time.

Outside investors understood that the extreme economic pressure created an opportunity for corporations to capture dentists, similar to how pharmacists were captured 40 years earlier.[44] But what they didn't understand was the significant difference between the practice of dentistry and the practice of pharmacy. Pharmacy is a very objective profession, whereas dentistry, at its highest level, is both right-brain and left-brain, objective and subjective, precise and creative, as well as relationship-driven. Consequently, most dentists don't like to be micromanaged, as they want to be free to exercise their best judgment and skills at the appropriate times.

Job dissatisfaction caused by corporatization has subsequently led to more and more transient relationships between dentists and employers, with the outcome being fewer stable, long-term relationships between dentists and their patients. For example, a practice in my community purchased by a corporation, has had four different dentists working in it over the past three years. The patients of the original practice are confused and are leaving. The dentist, who died of cancer, would be very distressed if he knew how his patients are being treated as if they were a commodity to be manipulated for financial gain.

I cringe at the thought of the size of some dentists' loan payments, and therefore, how much they need each patient. When we put ourselves into a situation where we need patients more than they need us, we are going to have a communication problem right out of the gate.

~Robert F. Barkley, D.D.S. (*A Preventive-Corrective Approach*, Emory University Dental School Presentation, 1973)

Chapter 12
Taylorism And Health Care

Frederick Taylor (1856–1915) was an American mechanical engineer with a passion for discovering better ways to increase production efficiency. He was one of the first management consultants in the United States and the originator of the terms Taylorism and the Rational Goal Model.[45]

Management is the process of achieving both individual and collective goals through the deployment and allocation of resources and decision-making. Its goals are achieved through improved performance, efficiency, innovation, and value creation. Frederick Taylor's Rational Goal Model trains managers to use science and analysis to achieve more effective outcomes and maximize profits:[46]

Identify the best way to perform an activity.

1. Select the best person to do the task (match person to the task).
2. Train that person to become optimally proficient at that task.
3. Link financial compensation to the performance of the task.
4. Centralize management of all tasks (top-down).

The outcome of Taylorism is fragmentation and micromanagement—complex processes are broken down into tasks which are optimized and timed as *efficiency is king.*

Taylor's ideas caught the attention of Henry Ford, and together they reduced production times and costs to a degree that Ford could lower prices and significantly increase profits. The increased profits allowed Ford to increase worker compensation, which caused the Detroit economy to boom. For the first time, Ford's workers could afford to buy the cars they built. Additionally, they bought small lake cottages, boats, and modest homes. But there was a problem inherent to the Rational Goal Model—it required workers to surrender their creative sovereignty; It required them to be used like robots. Better pay and a higher standard of living were traded for mindless repetition and feeling devalued as a person.

Newton's Third Law is "For every action, there is an equal and opposite reaction,"—and that's what happened next. Labor unions formed to fight against the working conditions overseen by technocratic managers focused on kinematics. The mind of a technocrat is preoccupied with the need to control outcomes, combined with a general distrust of worker motivations and behavior. Manufacturing cars, which had previously been a cooperative venture, evolved into an *us* versus *them* scenario, as employees were dehumanized to meet production goals.

The principles of Taylorism are now firmly entrenched in the healthcare industry, and are triggering similar unionization threats. The reason you rarely speak to a pharmacist is Taylorism. The reason your PCP is only allowed eight minutes in an examination room is Taylorism.[47] Taylorism is the reason why you see a physical therapy assistant instead of a physical therapist, and why insurance companies pay you a low wage for piecemeal work. How can a practice that's dependent upon insurance company reimbursement successfully function today?—by employing more Taylorism through more analysis and micromanagement.

The impact of Taylorism eventually led me into a conversation with a ten-year veteran hygienist who said, "I thought that I was entering a profession that was focused on helping people. Now, I feel like a production worker who is being encouraged to push products and procedures just to meet practice production goals." She told me that she was planning to leave the profession after completion of her bachelor's degree.

Corporate dentists are similarly managed and subsequently come and go at corporate practices after their creative spirits have been drained.[48] What are sincerely caring dentists, hygienists, and other dental team members supposed to do in a world full of Taylorism?

Chapter 13
The 23 Characteristics Of Tier III Practices

The corporatization trend is in direct conflict with the ever-advancing capabilities of today's dentistry. Additionally, it has created a gap between what employers and the insurance industry offer and what many people need and want. The highly personalized Tier III practice model is intended to address health-centered market trends. Consequently, those who understand how the Tier III practice model works are in an ideal position to successfully engage a growing market segment of people who are more likely to request our best and finest services, in addition to collaborating with us on long-range, health-centered goals.

As I have worked with my care team in addition to many others who transitioned to Tier III, I identified 23 common characteristics:

1. **Tier III practices are visionary**. The creation of a practice vision by a Tier III dentist represents an act of optimism. At the core of that optimism is faith – faith in their ability to adapt and create a practice of choice. The vision is a natural outgrowth of clarified core values, principles, and desires, and it's used by the dentist-leader to select and develop a care team that's capable of attracting patients who align well with those principles and values.

2. **Tier III practices have a clear Mission.** A practice mission is related to *how* the philosophy-inspired vision is implemented on a daily basis. Much like a practice vision, a mission is unique and values/principles-centered. A Tier III mission is collaboratively developed, nurtured, implemented, and routinely refined by the entire care team.

3. **Tier III practices utilize the power of synergy.** Tier III dentists know that team synergy catapults a practice to new heights. Conversely, a team that lacks the power of synergy substantially undermines the practice's performance. Therefore, Tier III dentists view team-building as a top priority as it fosters growth, collaborative interaction, and optimal outcomes.

4. **Tier III practices are committed to maintaining advanced clinical skills.** The Tier III dentist and care team take their professional development very seriously. They view constant refinement of their clinical skills and knowledge as an essential part of their role as leaders.

5. **Tier III practices are committed to mastering interpersonal skills.** The dentist and care team recognize that clinical mastery alone isn't enough to achieve consistent long-term practice success. They view dentistry as being both technical and behavioral, and subsequently facilitate values clarification, problem identification, ownership, appropriate choice-making, and collaboration.

6. **Tier III practices are committed to "organizational wellness."** Successful Tier III practices recognize that sustained, meaningful service to others requires that the emotional and financial needs of those who work within the practice are also being met. Consequently, Tier III practices are, at their core, emotionally and financially secure businesses capable of keeping the needs of their patients first-in-mind. Organizational wellness creates emotional and financial strength that's used strategically to avoid situations wherein the practice's financial needs might interfere with how, when, and why a patient is being treated.

7. **Tier III practices have successfully integrated laboratory functions**. Tier III practices recognize that the dental laboratory staff is an integral part of the total care team. They understand that it's the dentist's responsibility to have a working knowledge of all laboratory processes so they can assume a well-informed leadership role with laboratory technicians. The Tier III dentist willingly assumes full accountability to the patient for the quality of all dental work provided. That commitment to quality is widely known and frequently cited as why many patients choose to enter and stay with the practice.

8. **Tier III practices provide care within an appropriately designed facility.** Tier III practices have a facility that demonstrates planned excellence. By design, Tier III facilities support personal and professional growth, by making it easier to render out the finest care and services to their patients. Tier III facilities are also unique and represent the care team's commitment to quality. The design of the facility fosters a smooth flow of technical tasks and interpersonal relationships. As a result, Tier III facilities support privacy, respect, comfort, sincere caring, and personalized attention.

9. **Tier III practices have mastered health-centered relationship marketing skills.** Tier III teams recognize that fine dental care isn't designed for the "income elite" but for those who value dental health highly and see it as an essential part of their total wellness. A Tier III practice understands who these people are, what they want, and how to create and maintain long-term collaborative working relationships.

10. **Tier III practices have developed supportive practice systems**. Well-designed practice management systems exist to ensure that the practice's mission is smoothly executed on a daily basis. Many of the dysfunctional medical model

systems, that are reactive and unit-oriented (and which overtly or subliminally imply to patients that the primary objective of the practice is to make money), have been replaced by wellness model systems, that nurture health, sustainability, and patient self-responsibility. The care team's mission helps define the practice systems, which are measured and monitored by the care team.

11. **Tier III practices are committed to the development of leadership skills.** The Tier III dentist understands that when they lead the care team to share ownership of the practice vision and mission, they have successfully empowered the organization. The Tier III dentist understands that real leadership power is achieved through the empowerment of others. A dentist who exhibits a high level of leadership power can be viewed as a person to whom the care team has given the gift of reciprocal empowerment through their faith in their ability to lead them toward win-win scenarios.

12. **Similarly, the dentist can more easily lead patients toward,** more optimal health choices through their effective communication and teaching abilities. For many Tier III dentists, their leadership extends out beyond their practice into study clubs, dental societies, faculty positions, and mentoring.

13. **Tier III practices demonstrate emotional intelligence.** Tier III dentists exhibit a high level of emotional maturity. Emotional maturity includes self-awareness, self-regulation, motivation, empathy, and social skills. The dentist selects for and nurtures, emotional maturity within the care team as well. High levels of emotional intelligence support self-confidence and a willingness to take risks for the benefit of positive change. Self-confidence and willingness to take risks are core components of creativity, an ever-present force within a successful Tier III practice.

14. Tier III practices favor a multi-disciplinary approach to care. The Tier III dentist has nurtured and developed strong collaborative relationships with dental and medical specialists in the vicinity of their practice. It's noteworthy that these specialists have a high level of trust and faith in the care, skill, and judgment of the Tier III dentist and vice versa.

15. Tier III practices master clinical photography. Tier III practitioners consistently exhibit a high level of clinical photography skills. Those skills are frequently used for patient education, case documentation, group consultations, and presentations.

16. Tier III practices have health-centered hygiene departments. Tier III practices have successfully transitioned away from the traditional insurance-driven, high-volume hygiene practice model. The success of their hygiene department is less measured by productivity (although they are highly productive) than by the health, and movement toward health, of the patients within it. Those outcomes are achieved through exceptional clinical skills and collaborative relationship-building skills within the hygiene team.

17. Tier III practices understand communication styles and how people learn. Tier III practices are masterful at consistently facilitating their patients' awareness of their current dental health status through experiential learning. Tier III practices have an enhanced understanding of *how* people learn, and therefore are able to individualize the learning process for each person. The care team helps each patient to clarify their value for dental health, while they assist each person in the process of making better decisions.

18. **Tier III practices "walk the talk."** The Tier III practice demonstrates a high level of congruence between what it says it believes and what it does on a day-to-day basis. Thus, practice authenticity is the outcome of a shared commitment to the vision and mission by the entire team.

19. **Tier III practices demonstrate an unwavering commitment to professionalism.** The practice exhibits true professionalism, which in action is similar to the meaning of the Greek word for love, *agape*, and defined as a willingness to selflessly put the best interests of others ahead of one's own interests for the purpose of growth and development.

20. **Tier III practices are balanced.** The structure and systems of a Tier III practice allow for an uncommon balance between Work, Play, Love, and Worship. Tier III dentists consistently exhibit healthy interpersonal relationships with their family, team, patients, friends, colleagues, and community.

21. **Tier III practices are spiritual and sharing.** Tier III dentists understand, "Of those to whom much is given, much is expected." They also understand the value of two meaningful gifts: creativity and a sense of humor. These gifts help us to achieve our highest aspirations while simultaneously helping us to cope with our humanness along the way. Tier III dentists also understand the value of reflecting and drawing upon the strength of a higher purpose.

22. **Tier III practices masterfully manage patient expectations.** Tier III practices are very adept at clear, concise communication with their patients. They have well-designed patient education materials and policy guidelines that function seamlessly with planned discussions regarding the practice philosophy, financial obligations, scheduling policies, and home care responsibilities. Therefore, Tier III

practices experience few misunderstandings regarding money, compliance, insurance company actions, and scheduling. Additionally, they are adept at communicating with patients via the use of diagnostic wax-ups, approved provisional restorations, and photography.

23. Tier III practices prefer the lower-volume, higher-profitability practice model. Tier III practices recognize that a well-managed smaller practice is consistently more successful at optimizing patient health than a well-managed large practice. That outcome is due to the synergistic effect of relationships unique to smaller, more personalized environments. Tier III dentists also acknowledge that successful, fine dentistry is as much a creative act as it is a highly technical one, and that consistently high levels of creativity are only possible when sufficient time is allowed for it to occur.

24. Tier III practices abandon trying to be everything to everyone. They believe that such a strategy dilutes limited resources and ultimately the quality of outcomes over time. Instead, Tier III practices focus their attention on excellence through the use of personalized care strategies. Tier III practices properly price their services so that they are an accurate reflection of their care, skill, and judgment.

25. Tier III practices function independently of the needs of the insurance industry. Tier III practices have successfully transitioned away from being dependent on insurance industry reimbursement patterns. The goal is achieved through building patient appreciation for their practice philosophy, combined with CoDiscovery, controlled overhead expenses, and the termination of provider contracts with insurance carriers.

The benefits of achieving independence from negative insurance industry influence are multi-fold:

1. It helps reinforce the practice's mission to provide primarily comprehensive, health-centered restorative services.

2. It removes the insurance industry's agendas from the treatment planning process and properly focuses the patient's attention on their preferred long-term outcome and how to best achieve it.

3. It fosters financial self-responsibility on the part of the patient.

4. It unburdens the practice from real or perceived accountability to third parties.

5. It returns ownership of the actions of insurance companies to the employers and subscribers.

6. It allows the practice to accurately set fees that are reflective of the true value of services provided.

7. It allows the practice to focus on the most appropriate care instead of being enslaved to a least expensive alternative care orientation.

8. It helps protect a practice's financial future through the elimination of the insurance industry's ability to manipulate fees, profit margins, patient flow, or the withholding of a significant amount of rightfully earned income.

9. It allows for more time to develop genuine helping relationships with each person and to avoid the hollow, task-oriented encounters that are frequently the outgrowth of fast-paced, insurance-dependent practices.

Chapter 14
The Tier III Checklist

1. I have a written practice Philosophy Statement that's clarified down to fit on one page.

   Strongly Disagree   1 2 3 4 5 6 7 8 9 10   Strongly Agree

2. I have a clear Vision in my mind of what my ideal practice looks, feels, and functions like.

   Strongly Disagree   1 2 3 4 5 6 7 8 9 10   Strongly Agree

3. I have a clarified Mission, my philosophy in action, that will lead me to my vision.

   Strongly Disagree   1 2 3 4 5 6 7 8 9 10   Strongly Agree

4. I have selected and developed a *care team* that functions at a high level of *synergy.*

   Strongly Disagree   1 2 3 4 5 6 7 8 9 10   Strongly Agree

5. I have learned and mastered the *clinical skills* necessary to achieve my Vision.

   Strongly Disagree   1 2 3 4 5 6 7 8 9 10   Strongly Agree

6. My care team has developed the interpersonal skills necessary to achieve my Vision.

   Strongly Disagree   1 2 3 4 5 6 7 8 9 10   Strongly Agree

7. My practice is financially stable, which allows me to keep my patient's needs ahead of my own.

   Strongly Disagree   1 2 3 4 5 6 7 8 9 10   Strongly Agree

8. I have successfully integrated critical laboratory functions, and my facility is designed in such a way that I am able to accomplish lab work in a comfortable, organized fashion.

   Strongly Disagree 1 2 3 4 5 6 7 8 9 10 Strongly Agree

9. I work within a properly designed facility that optimally supports my mission.

   Strongly Disagree 1 2 3 4 5 6 7 8 9 10 Strongly Agree

10. I know my target ideal clients, and know how to communicate with them via marketing.

   Strongly Disagree 1 2 3 4 5 6 7 8 9 10 Strongly Agree

11. My practice management systems run smoothly, and predictably support my practice mission.

   Strongly Disagree 1 2 3 4 5 6 7 8 9 10 Strongly Agree

12. I understand and deploy *principle-centered leadership skills* that consistently help me to advance my practice mission toward my vision.

   Strongly Disagree 1 2 3 4 5 6 7 8 9 10 Strongly Agree

13. We demonstrate emotional intelligence every day.

   Strongly Disagree 1 2 3 4 5 6 7 8 9 10 Strongly Agree

14. I believe in the value of a multi-disciplinary approach to care, and have established trusting, collaborative relationships with my specialists and medical community peers.

   Strongly Disagree 1 2 3 4 5 6 7 8 9 10 Strongly Agree

15. I have mastered clinical photography for the purpose of examination, communication, presentations, and proper documentation.

Strongly Disagree 1 2 3 4 5 6 7 8 9 10 Strongly Agree

16. I have a health-centered hygiene department, wherein health is effectively promoted and very little remedial work is required on patients who regularly participate in the practice.

Strongly Disagree 1 2 3 4 5 6 7 8 9 10 Strongly Agree

17. My care team understands how people learn and manages education on the individual level (instead of in a standardized fashion) to optimize the communication of important information, support clarification of values and priorities, and better decision-making.

Strongly Disagree 1 2 3 4 5 6 7 8 9 10 Strongly Agree

18. My practice "walks the talk." We are who we say we are. We are congruent philosophically and on the mission level.

Strongly Disagree 1 2 3 4 5 6 7 8 9 10 Strongly Agree

19. We generally lead balanced lives, and when one of us is confronted with a challenge or a situation that pushes our life out of balance, we do everything possible to help them out. Thus, we act as a unified caring, supportive, values-centric community.

Strongly Disagree 1 2 3 4 5 6 7 8 9 10 Strongly Agree

20. My practice is spiritual and sharing, as we all believe, "Of those to whom much is given, much is expected." Thus, we approach each day with gratitude and demonstrate genuine caring and love.

Strongly Disagree   1 2 3 4 5 6 7 8 9 10   Strongly Agree

21. We consistently manage expectations on a high level with regard to how the treatment process will go, in addition to financial and other responsibilities.

Strongly Disagree   1 2 3 4 5 6 7 8 9 10   Strongly Agree

22. Functionally, we run a lower-volume, high-profitability per-patient business model.

Strongly Disagree   1 2 3 4 5 6 7 8 9 10   Strongly Agree

23. My practice is largely free of the negative influence of insurance companies.

Strongly Disagree   1 2 3 4 5 6 7 8 9 10   Strongly Agree

Dentists don't compete against other dentists, they compete against realtors, car dealers, travel agents, and others who provide discretionary services people truly desire. The problem today is not that there are too many dentists, rather there are too few people who are at a point where they value dentistry and dental health highly enough to make the sacrifices to pursue it.

The challenge ahead for the dental profession is to figure out how to leave the medical model behind, which only remedies deficiencies, and move on to develop a more health-centered model in which people grow and develop greater value for more comprehensive help and relationships. In this new and emerging model, dentistry is a means for facilitating health rather than just an end unto itself.

I believe that dentistry is coming into its greatest years, but only for dentists who use creative management skills and who are able to acknowledge that health is not so much about the complete absence of disease, but rather is a quality of life which is independent of disease.

~Avrom E. King, M.S.

Dental Economics (May 1980)

One question, one answer, and I knew immediately that I shouldn't even touch her. I would have never been able to do that, if I had not met L.D. Pankey. So, what I am trying to tell you here, is that the new patient interview matters more than you will ever know. But, just like many of you, when I first heard L. D. speak on this topic, I totally missed the value of it. Six months later, however, I realized that it was something that I desperately needed to understand if I wanted to become more successful.

~F. Harold Wirth, D.D.S.

Audio recording of L. D. Pankey, Denver, CO (1986)

Chapter 15
F. Harold Wirth, D.D.S.

It's virtually impossible to have a conversation about the life of L.D. Pankey without including a discussion of his relationship with F. Harold Wirth. Harold started his practice in New Orleans, just before The Great Depression. He would go on to develop a very successful restorative practice and speaking career, but like most dentists, it didn't start out that way. According to Harold, it was only after he realized "that dentistry was about a lot more than just teeth," that things started to change for the better.

Harold took Dale Carnegie courses and read Norman Vincent Peale, in addition to many other authors, to help refine his communication skills. He also learned how to speed-read, which allowed him to consume a book a day. Over time, Harold's reading habits caused his personal library to grow so large that it was donated to the LSU Dental School library after his passing. The collection includes books on psychology, communication, writing, public speaking, motivation, positive mental attitude, and much more.[49]

On the clinical development side, Harold completed a post-graduate year in restorative dentistry at the University of Toronto, working under the leadership of Harold Box, a protégé of Dr. Gotlieb of Vienna, Austria. As a result, Harold said, "If you had asked me if I knew anything about occlusion, I would have said 'yes,' because that was where I was first exposed to the concept of equilibration and methods of stabilizing teeth via what they were calling periodontal membrane re-attachment."[50]

Harold heard Dr. Pankey speak for the first time at a presentation to his study group at the Roosevelt Hotel in 1955. At that time, Harold was under the impression that Dr. Pankey's expertise was primarily related to group practice management, as he had successfully led a multi-doctor practice in Coral Gables, Florida, for decades. Harold soon realized, however, that Dr. Pankey had a much bigger message to share. He said, "After listening to Dr. Pankey for two days, a door opened for me. I was able to see a vista of what dentistry *could be*, a perspective that I didn't think existed, and I knew that it was something that I wanted to do."[51]

Prior to that time, Harold said that his practice was financially successful and busy, "My operatories were so duplicated that every instrument was the same, and I practiced like a lion in a cage with my head down...I went back and forth, back and forth...I don't think I ever saw a patient, I just saw teeth and dentistry." He described his situation as a "rut" that was getting deeper. Harold knew that the only way out was to "pull hard on the wheel and keep pulling, or I'd just slip right back into it."[52]

Dr. Pankey's presentation put a thought in Harold's mind that would eventually liberate him from that rut, in addition to making significant improvements to his personal health habits. Harold carefully took notes and studied the manual, "I studied it and I studied it, until I was sure that I understood it." Then, Harold began the process of applying the concepts while staying in contact with Dr. Pankey. "I would occasionally call L.D. and say, *You would have been really proud of me today!—or I'd say to myself, that's exactly what he told me to do!—or I really flubbed that one up! L.D. would have kicked me in the behind if he had been hanging over my shoulder that day!*"[53]

Harold Wirth was such a good student and practitioner of L.D. Pankey's concepts, which Dr. Pankey gave him permission to speak to Pankey Study Groups. Harold said, "I always carried around that manual, it was practically worn out after repeatedly thumbing through it...You had to live the philosophy vividly, and understand it so thoroughly that it becomes a part of you—and at that point, you become comfortable with all of it."[54]

In 1958, L.D. Pankey asked Harold to join him to teach *The Philosophy* around the world. That partnership would continue up until Harold's passing in 1987. In March of that year, Harold was moderating a meeting of the New Orleans Dental Association, when the topics of entrepreneurship, PPOs, and marketing were discussed. As Harold called the meeting to a close, everyone could see that he was visibly upset when he said, *"I didn't hear anyone say anything about how we can take better care of our patients, nor did I didn't hear a single person mention the word love. There will always be free enterprise, private practice for the caring dentist who seeks excellence for their patients through the exercise of the greatest skill and judgment at their command. For those who are concerned, don't worry – they will seek you out. End of story. No rebuttal."*

As Harold descended from the podium, he fell into the arms of Dr. Mike Robichaux, while suffering a fatal heart attack. Mike later said, "My life changed forever at that moment." [55]

Chapter 16
Richard A. Green, DDS, MBA

If you have been to The Pankey Institute, you are familiar with Rich Green and his legacy.[56] Rich grew up in Hinsdale, a western suburb of Chicago. Rich met Dr. John A. Anderson in 1956 while he was in high school during a church event. John was a pioneer and an innovator who would go on to help create The Pankey Institute in 1970. Rich said that John was a "boundary pusher," who was committed to continuing his development throughout his life—a mindset Rich soon adopted.

After high school, Rich attended North Park College, close to John Anderson's office, and where he was able to observe and further develop his interest in dentistry. Rich then attended Northwestern's School of Dentistry, graduating in 1966. He practiced in Hinsdale after completing of a residency program at Denver General Hospital. Rich said, "Starting out in my career, I felt well-trained technically, yet I must have subtly believed that I was a 'hardware salesperson' because I found it easier to talk 'hardware and technique' than to listen well and help my patients clarify their health objectives."

The "hardware" selling stage of Rich's career was short-lived after meeting both L.D. Pankey and Bob Barkley in 1968. John Anderson encouraged Rich to fly down to Florida and attend a two-and-a-half-day PMS/Oral Rehabilitation Seminar. Additionally, a local Pankey study group known as the "Pankey Prophets" invited Rich to join them in Williamsburg, Virginia where Dr. Pankey was speaking. That same year, Rich's transported Bob Barkley from the local airport to help him prepare to give a presentation that included his 5-day disease control program. Bob was extroverted, funny, and confident. According to Rich, Bob was less concerned about *what* people learned than *how* they were going to apply it, so he spent most of the day discussing the philosophy of learning, while frequently referencing *The Age of Discontinuity*, a new book written by Peter Drucker. The actual step-by-step process of Bob's prevention program only took him an hour to explain. In today's terms, Bob was focused on the "why" and not just the "what," because he knew that if the dentists didn't buy into the philosophy *behind the how,* they would fail to successfully apply the information and then blame him for wasting time and money.

Bob was an avid student of *learning about how people learn*, a passion heavily influenced by Nate Kohn, Jr. Rich soon adopted a similar interest that carried him through the next twenty-five years of private practice, teaching at The Pankey Institute as an original Cadre' member, a fourteen-year association with Don Clifton and The Gallup Organization (encouraged by Bob Barkley), the creation of the Pankey Patient and Team Satisfaction Surveys, the completion of an MBA, the creation and direction of Business Systems Development at The Pankey Institute, running a practice consultancy, and extensive writing.

Rich was 25 when he first met Dr. Pankey, and they would grow to become good friends. When Rich combined what he learned from Dr. Pankey with that of Bob Barkley, it catalyzed within him the need to pursue additional knowledge from Carl Rogers, Chuck Sorensen, Don Clifton, Henry Tanner, Avrom King, and many others.

As a student of Rich Green, I learned about The Three Riddles: Technical, Behavioral, and Communication, all of which demand constant attention, learning, re-assessment, and application by the process of putting them into "the crucible," – our subconscious, values-driven decision-making process. Rich said:

Each patient who sits in your chair has at least three riddles that you can begin to understand and address. If the patient would like to have the greatest potential for keeping his or her teeth for a lifetime and to optimize health, function, and aesthetics, you can begin to learn, understand, and address all three.

In an article titled *Learning About Learning*, Rich wrote:

In a uniquely individualized, relationship-based, values-driven, fee-for-service practice, which promotes positive health choices, time is allowed to help the patient clarify his or her best choices while connecting those choices to his or her expressed values…In these uniquely individualized collaborations, we can learn to facilitate a new awareness of health and to develop an awareness that helps to transfer the locus of control back to the patient. When we can accomplish this ownership transfer back to the patient, the outcome is that all stakeholders increase their own awareness and health through healthier behaviors and boundaries.

Chapter 17
What Does a Person-Centered Practice Look Like?

Dr. Frederico Lima was trained in postgraduate prosthodontics in both Brazil and the United States, but that's not what makes him special. What makes Fred stand out is his exceptional ability to connect with people, help them learn what they need to know about proper, comprehensive, health-centered dentistry, and then facilitate better decision-making. The following is one story of many similar experiences:

Tom was referred to me by a patient who thought that I would be able to help. Tom was initially interviewed by Jennifer, my patient care coordinator, in my consultation room. The interview was unexpectedly short, leading Jennifer to prematurely enter my private office and say, "Tom is ready to see you, but I need to warn you that he just told me that he isn't interested in a comprehensive examination or willing to allow us to take any radiographs."

I took a deep breath and wondered what was going on. After all, Tom was referred by a great patient. I entered the consultation room and introduced myself. Over the years, I've noticed that almost everyone is comfortable talking about themselves, so I used that strategy to break the tension in the room. "It's great to meet you, Tom, are you a Texas native?" Tom told me that he grew up in California, so I asked, "I have a good friend that grew up in California as well. What part are you from?" My intention was to move Tom's mind away from his apprehension and onto a topic that he was more comfortable discussing—my goal was also to get him to see me as a caring person and not as just another indifferent dentist entering his life. I knew that if I could achieve those goals, he'd be more prone to telling me why he was opposed to allowing an examination and x-rays.

After discussing where Tom grew up, I started to gain a better sense of who he was, as it led him to share his passion for American history. As that conversation unfolded, it was clear to me that Tom was very bright and self-disciplined. He also possessed a driven, curious mind that paid a lot of attention to small details.

Over the years, I've taught myself to avoid making too many assumptions about people because, in almost every case, when I create the opportunity for a person to share a little bit more about themselves, the conversation will turn in an unexpected direction and I learn something that helps me to connect on a deeper level. For example, a person's chief complaint is often not their primary issue, it's often a symptom of a much bigger problem that they don't know exists. Most of us weren't trained to be effective interviewers, but it's one of the most important skills that I've mastered, as it's frequently the only way to understand a person's problems from their perspective.

Tom was very articulate, much like a person playing a masterful guitar solo, as he created a narrative that flowed along nicely. He eventually told me why he decided to call my office: A good friend told him, "Dr. Lima has a more holistic way of working with people." Now, I have to say that up until that moment, I'd never thought of myself as being a "holistic" dentist, but the way Tom explained it to me, it made perfect sense—so I embraced it. To Tom, holistic meant *comprehensive, systematic, and highly integrated*. He was a mechanical engineer who viewed everything as being part of an integrated system, all the way up to his relationship with God.

Tom went on to discuss a career that had led him to participate in projects all over the world. He told me that he'd finally reached the point in his life where he was ready to slow down and focus more of his time and attention on consulting and speaking. But there was one problem with his plan: His teeth were discolored, worn down, and crooked, so Tom didn't look good in photographs, in corporate conference rooms, during video conferences, or when he was up at the podium. In other words, Tom was embarrassed about his appearance. Tom knew his dental system was a mess, and he didn't want others to know about it—that's what appealed to Tom when he heard about Fred, the 'holistic" dentist. But he was also scared, because none of his previous dentists had ever taken the time to listen to his concerns or to work with him in a way that made sense to his highly analytical mind. As a result, he responded defensively: "I don't want any x-rays or a complete examination."

I told Tom that I could successfully address his problems in an organized, systematic, and predictable fashion. I also told him that the development of a successful plan was only possible after a survey of his current condition on both the physical and functional levels, including radiographs. I said, "Just like an engineer approaches the creation of a technical design proposal, we need to do some research and analysis before we develop a plan, which includes a careful study of the condition of your teeth, bite, gums, jawbone structure, and jaw joint function. All of those areas need to be evaluated separately as well as together because they are all part of a very complex and highly integrated system."

As I explained the value of a proper examination to Tom, he nodded his head without saying a word. It was easily apparent to him that a successful plan of action hinged off on accurate analysis, something that he'd been doing as an engineer for over thirty years. At that point, Tom agreed to allow a full series of radiographs, photographs, and other preliminary records, which were completed that day after my muscle and joint evaluation. During those processes, I talked about the value of co-developing a plan that would improve his smile and the appearance of his teeth. By the end of the visit, Tom was acting like a different person, his personality had opened up and he was much more conversational. On his way out, we shook hands as he told me that he was looking forward to his next appointment.

Before that visit, I organized my photographs, mounted and analyzed the study casts, and put together some teaching aids so that I would be able to clarify some important points. When Tom arrived, I took him through the photographs, radiographs, and study models while asking him questions that strategically engaged his analytical mind. Once Tom was more familiar with how his mouth looked in photographs, radiographs, and study models, we headed back to the operatory to complete the CoDiscovery examination. As important findings were discovered, I referenced what we had reviewed and discussed in the consultation room, and then correlated it to what we were seeing in the mouth. Tom commented, "I think we are moving in the right direction." CoDiscovery is the vehicle through which all of the above can happen, however, it's only possible when we're willing to take the time to listen from a place of non-judgment, and with no intention to manipulate the outcome. That's important, because people sense danger when they are being "sold." Healthcare shouldn't be about sales; rather, it should be centered around effective teaching that leads to better decision-making. Sir William Osler, the father of modern medicine, said:

You are in this profession as a calling, not as a business—a calling, which exacts from you at every turn self-sacrifice, devotion, and love and tenderness to your fellow man. Once you get down to a purely business level, your influence is gone, and the true light of your life is dimmed. You must work in the missionary spirit, with a breadth of charity that rises you far above the petty jealousies of life.

Upon the completion of the second appointment, I asked Tom if he wanted me to assemble a comprehensive plan that addressed all of the issues we had discussed, as well as the creation of a long-lasting, stable, and attractive smile. He said that he was very interested in seeing a comprehensive plan, and that my examination process was by far the most careful and complete evaluation he had ever experienced. His response was *exactly* what I wanted to hear. Tom said that today's world is full of information, but the challenge is that most information has yet to be translated into practical knowledge. He went on to explain the difference between knowledge and the acquisition of wisdom, and that we must learn how to apply our knowledge in a wise fashion, a statement that made me think about L.D. Pankey's *Cross of Dentistry*.

Tom also mentioned the pioneering work of E. Edwards Deming and his Total Quality Management concept, commonly referred to as TQM. Tom felt that Deming's work was directly applicable to dentistry. I was pleased to know that Tom was comfortable talking to me as a friend and not just as a dentist. I wanted to understand why Tom felt TQM was so important, because later that day, he texted a screenshot showing a graphic of Deming's 14-point philosophy along with the statement, "Personalize it!"

Tom was challenging me to grow, so I purchased the book *The World of W. Edwards Deming*. When Tom arrived for the next appointment, he was surprised to learn that I was prepared to discuss Deming. Jennifer escorted him into the consultation room, where mounted master casts were situated alongside a beautiful diagnostic wax-up that my wife had prepared. The "before" and "after" models functioned as a perfect representation of what was possible for him. Jennifer left Tom alone in the room for a few minutes, to allow time for his analytical mind to kick into gear. As expected, when I entered, Tom was excited about the projected outcome, and he wanted to know more about how it could be achieved. Up until that moment, Tom had never had the opportunity to envision what his mouth would look like if it was strategically restored. As I explained each step, Tom interrupted me, completed my sentences, and then elaborated on his understanding by using engineering terminology. At that point, I was all smiles, as it was clear to me that CoDiscovery had allowed Tom to understand what the treatment meant to him. In other words, Tom's understanding had reached a level that he no longer needed me to function as his savior, instead he wanted to partner with me on a very important project.

Jennifer was mesmerized by Tom's desire to take the lead and collaborate on the creation of an optimal solution. I said, "Tom, I'm thinking of asking you to join me in this practice as a partner instead of just allowing you to be a patient. You not only understand everything on the technical level, but you also have a lot to teach me!" We laughed, but I was partly serious, as I always learn something when I listen carefully. Tom appreciated that I'd taken the time to "personalize it."

This type of interaction is very familiar to me. I have learned over the years that there are many different versions of "Tom" out there, and that I will only find them when I intentionally create an environment that allows them to appear. As I progressively learned more and more about how to do that, my practice changed for the better. I believe that your practice can change as well if you simply follow the principles outlined in this book.

In my early professional years, I would have asked the question: How can I treat, cure, or change this person? Now, I would phrase the question this way: How can I provide a relationship which this person may use for their own personal growth?"

~Carl R. Rogers, PhD

On Becoming a Person, Harper One, 2nd ed., 1950, p. 26

Chapter 18
Bob Barkley's Connection to Carl Rogers

ob Barkley said:

Carl Rogers stated that the only learning which significantly influences behavior is self-appropriated learning, yet few examinations are arranged so that the patient learns with the doctor… [When self-appropriated learning is not part of the process,] the doctor must 'teach' the patient his examination findings, and may support their teaching with various teaching aids. But significant learning takes place when the examination and the diagnosis time is shared by the dentist and patient…Patients can't listen to a barrage of explanations, while they are simultaneously thinking about how their dental health has affected, and will affect, their life in the future. Their belief in the value of a long-term preventive/ restorative solution therefore, can only be developed through inductive thinking – not through our explanations.*[57]

**Inductive thinking* is right-brain synthesis-oriented thinking that's used to tackle new challenges versus decision-making that's rather thoughtless and primarily based upon memory. We will discuss inductive thinking in more detail later in this book, as it's key to understanding how people tend to make complex decisions.

Do you feel good after the completion of a long conversation with someone who knows you well on an emotional level? That's because, those types of conversations cause us to feel more positive and hopeful. When a person gifts us their full attention and simultaneously makes no attempt to judge, we tend to share more feelings, which leads us into a deeper level of self-understanding and acceptance.

Carl Rogers took the common elements of truly helping relationships and applied them to his work as a psychologist and counselor. The outcome was a new way to help others make significant changes in their lives. Along the way, his concepts challenged historical doctor-patient relationship models.[58]

Rogers, who had a doctorate in psychology from Columbia University, graduated with the assumption that his counseling skills were good enough to solve most of the problems he would see in practice. He soon realized however, that his treatment approaches weren't successful with the patients who needed the most help. Rogers also noticed that sustainable positive change within a person was influenced more by the *quality* of the relationship than by the specific technique or strategy deployed by the therapist. Rogers noted that successful helping relationships had within them a philosophy that Martin Buber referred to as "confirmation the other"—the helper had a pattern of affirming the inherent value of the person as well as their potential for positive change. The "confirmation of the other" process was non-judgmental and allowed the person time to safely explore the possibility of a change in their perspective—a transformation of the way they thought about themselves and onward toward a realization that they had so much potential – a vision of "what they had been created to become."

The shift away from an emphasis on *what's wrong* (the Freudian approach) to a focus on *what's possible,* turned Rogers into a leader of a new movement called humanistic psychology. (When we fast forward fifty years, we see a lot of Carl Rogers ideas in the growth and development movements of Tony Robbins, Stephen Covey, and many others.)[59]

In his early training, Carl Rogers was taught to control the doctor-patient relationship, and that it was his responsibility to analyze and treat each person. However, Rogers discovered that when he did the opposite—when he let his adult clients guide the timing, direction, and nature of the treatment process, he was much more successful. Roger's new approach emphasized personal empowerment through active participation in the problem-solving process. He called the new approach *person-centered* therapy.

Carl Rogers began every relationship with active listening because it helped promote self-reflection. His goal was to understand how each person perceived their situation, what they believed caused it, how the problem was influencing their life, and what they wanted to do about it. Carl listened without judgment, even when the stories sounded unlikely or highly inaccurate. His approach functioned like a mirror, helping each person to see themselves more accurately—perhaps for the very first time.

Roger's approach was simple:

I'll try to be my authentic self while I withhold judgment, and let the other person reveal their true self to themselves. Then, we'll explore who they think they are, how they feel about it, and what changes they might want to make to improve their life.

Carl advanced his approach at the same time others were turning their attention to the theories of B. F. Skinner, who frequently compared human behavior to rats under experimental conditions—meaning that people are mostly reactionary and possess only a minimal amount of free will. Roger's philosophy—the belief that each person possesses a significant ability to initiate positive self-change, was counter-cultural. And if that wasn't enough, Carl challenged the belief that therapists should remain emotionally detached. Rogers felt that it was important for a therapist to understand their own feelings and to allow their instincts to play an emotionally intelligent role in the therapeutic process. He believed that an important aspect of trust-building included the helper appropriately revealing their personality and emotions within the therapeutic relationship at the right times—something he referred to as "genuineness." For example, if Carl Rogers felt sad or afraid during a session with a client, he would share his feelings by saying something like, "Hearing this really makes me feel sad," or "I can understand why that frightened you—just hearing about this frightens me too." Likewise, when Carl didn't have the answer to a particular problem, he wouldn't pretend that he did. Instead, he'd say something like, "At this point, I don't know what to say."

In sum, person-centered therapy[60] holds that significant change is best facilitated through a process that supports the development of more openness and honesty, and that it's the helper's responsibility to create an environment that allows it to evolve. Roger's felt life was a free-flowing process full of potentialities, and that satisfaction was most commonly found in people who were able to accept that life is a process, "a stream of becoming, and that the person is not a finished product."

Rogers observed that when people approached him for assistance, they would typically share a single reason why they thought they needed help, and that it was usually related to a conflict with their spouse, employer, family member, or an uncontrollable behavior pattern. But invariably, he'd discover that the problem was really just a symptom of a much bigger issue. Rogers noticed that each person eventually expressed a desire to live a more congruent life through a process of ridding themselves of dysfunctional roles, relationships, habits and masks. *"It seems that gradually, painfully, the individual explores what's behind the masks he presents to the world, and even behind the masks with which he has been deceiving himself... Thus, to an increasing degree, he becomes himself – not a facade of conformity to try and please others, not a cynical denial of all feeling, nor a front of intellectual rationality, but he becomes a living, breathing, feeling, fluctuating process - in short, he finally becomes a person.[61]*

Central to Rogers' philosophy was a belief that humans are "basically socialized, forward-moving, rational, and realistic," and that unproductive emotions are primarily a reflection of frustrations associated with not feeling loved, safe, successful, or accepted. He also believed that most people were capable of making good decisions with some level of facilitation.

How does Rogers' work relate to the practice of dentistry?

Bob Barkley became familiar with Carl Rogers' thinking through his close work with Nate Kohn, Jr., PhD. Over time, Bob developed ways to make his dental practice more "humanistic" through a belief that each person had the potential for a higher level of self-understanding that would eventually motivate positive self-change. Like Rogers, Bob's philosophy was counter-cultural relative to the consensus of that time, which was fatalistic and frequently something similar to: "My family has bad teeth. My fate is that I will lose some or all my teeth over my lifetime, so why should I make a big effort to change my current habits and perspective?" Bob wanted his patients to achieve a more optimal future through the establishment of a goal-oriented relationship that was centered around *their* values, priorities, and commitments.

Chapter 19
Michael Schuster, D.D.S.

Mike is a 1966 graduate of Marquette University School of Dentistry.[62] His father was a college professor and military strategic planner involved in the assault on Normandy Beach during World War II. He credits his father for exposing him to the writing of Abe Maslow and many other developmental thinkers.

Mike began practicing dentistry as a Navy Dental Corps officer at Willow Grove Naval Station, located north of Philadelphia. There, he became interested in conservative periodontal treatment and was allowed to take a five-day course at Walter Reed Army Medical Center. Bob Barkley spoke on the fourth day of that meeting, preceded by Harold Löe and several other leading voices in periodontics. "The seed was planted in my mind, and I started to question everything," Mike said.

After becoming the most productive and effective dentist at the Naval Station, and the completion of his service commitment, Mike set up a scratch practice in Dyersville, Iowa located in western Dubuque County, population 3,500. When Mike talks about that time in his life, his voice is full of emotion:

I got in trouble in Dyersville. I couldn't connect with people… I was able to pay off all of my school debt after working my way through dental school, but stress eventually landed me in the hospital at age 28 with a bleeding ulcer and the thought in my head that if that was what dentistry was all about, I'd have to find something else to do with my life.

Soon thereafter Mike called Bob Barkley, who lived less than 200 miles away. Mike felt that Bob likely had some answers because he practiced in a similar rural setting. Bob's response was, "Mike, there's nothing wrong with dentistry, but there is definitively something very wrong with the way you're practicing it."

Mike went on to fully integrate Bob Barkley's five-day Disease Control Program and then create his own version called "The Dental Fitness Program"[63] that closely tracked plaque levels, bleeding points, and diet for patients who were demonstrating active caries and periodontal disease. His program even helped patients balance their body chemistry via blood analysis and dietary changes. At its peak, Mike had two hygienists with master's degrees in nutrition, and all of his systems were computerized. Mike asked his patients: "How healthy and disease-free would you like to become?" After outgrowing his space, Mike moved his practice to Dubuque and then created a multi-specialty group with the assistance of Charles Sorensen; "As the patients became healthier, they'd ask me for more and more optimal care," Mike said.

A significant part of Mike's professional development was the result of his association with L.D. Pankey. Mike studied under Dr. Pankey prior to the inception of The Pankey Institute, and upon completion of the Continuum, was asked to be an instructor in 1974. Mike also enjoyed a close friendship with Harold Wirth, and would frequently travel to New Orleans to sail on Harold's boat and talk endlessly about the Institute, *The Philosophy,* the future, and current challenges.

Mike taught at The Pankey Institute for eleven years, and noticed that many dentists had money, tax, leadership and organizational problems. Those struggles catalyzed a desire to create a place where dentists could clarify their vision and master the leadership and management skills necessary to become successful at person-centered, health-centered dentistry. Mike's vision eventually evolved into *The Center for Professional Development,* an initiative that both Dr. Pankey and Dr. Wirth supported. Creation of the Center required Mike to sell his Dubuque practice, move to Phoenix, establish a new practice, and initially lead practice development workshops out of his living room.

After 11 years of contributing to The Pankey Institute, Mike shifted his full attention to the expansion of The Center, which enrolled 150-200 dentists per year at its peak. The curriculum was centered around practice management, disease control, philosophy, and other patient-centered services.

Mike said:

I dedicated my life to helping dentists help their patients in very profound ways. I've noticed over the years that the dentists who are the most successful at applying this kind of knowledge are those who are more spiritual – and I'm not talking about religion. They tend to use their life energy to help others, they are inherently more holistic – body, mind, spirit... The thing that really changed the course of my life was my health crisis at age 28. At that time, I was too focused on myself – my goals and what I wanted to do. That crisis forced me to transition away from an "it's about me" perspective to a "we" perspective, and that's made all the difference in the world on a number of levels.

When asked about who was most responsible for the major shift in his philosophy of practice, Mike said, "Bob Barkley and Dr. Pankey simultaneously affirmed the appropriateness of how I'd been raised."

Your time is limited, so don't waste it trying to live someone else's life.

~Steve Jobs

Commencement Address, Stanford University, 2005

Chapter 20
Why Is Trust Essential
To Every Helping Relationship?

Trust is commonly thought of as a firm belief in the reliability, truthfulness, and capability of another person, thing, or process. But in reality, trust is associated with vulnerability—how much vulnerability a person is willing to allow into their life at a particular point in time. So, the more a person trusts, the more they're willing to allow themselves to be potentially hurt; they make a risk-benefit analysis and decide to throw the dice.

Conversely, when a person isn't willing to trust, they have strategically decided to minimize their vulnerability. Thus, when a patient says *no* to x-rays, or to allowing us to proceed with a proper restoration, or other appropriate procedures, they're saying on a non-verbal level, "I don't trust you enough right now to allow you to do that." And when that occurs, it's easy for us to instinctively respond by projecting *our* values onto the situation. A better strategy is to empathetically explore *why* a person responded to the situation the way they did—try to understand the situation from *their* perspective, and then focus on finding common ground in shared goals and values (In Tom's case above, he wanted a more attractive, healthy smile but had no idea how to achieve that goal until Fred built a bridge of trust over to him, and then helped Tom to cross over and arrive at a place where more information was available and he could make *better* decisions). So, it's helpful to keep in mind *no* often means *not yet*, as in, "You haven't convinced me yet that I should allow myself to be that vulnerable around you."

Juxtaposed to our patients' level of trust *in us* is our trust *in them*. To do what Fred demonstrated with Tom required Fred to have a high level of trust in Tom's decision-making ability, which means that Fred was willing to invest time, energy, and money in the process of allowing Tom to learn more about his situation and choices, and then give Tom the time to make a decision based upon what he thought was in his best interest. So, CoDiscovery requires a leap of faith—a belief that most people will eventually do the right things for themselves. If you're unable to get yourself to a place where you can trust your patients on that level, then you're going to struggle with this practice model. Why? Because you'll tend to do what Fred used to do—you'll try to manipulate patients into doing what you want them to do, a behavior that drives emotionally sensitive patients away.

Our anxiety does not come from thinking about the future, but from our wanting to control it.

~Kahlil Gibran

Chapter 21
How to Build More Trusting Relationships

Trust represents our most valuable interpersonal currency, because without trust, we can't build the sustainable relationships we need to tackle complex problems. It's helpful to understand that there are two phases of trust: First, there's a *preconscious phase*, wherein the limbic system makes a security assessment. And it's only after this initial safety assessment is successfully completed, that a more conscious level of trust can evolve.

Regardless of what we'd like to achieve, our capacity to consistently build trust is central to our success. We're all wired for connection and to focus on ourselves and our "tribe." We want to feel significant, accepted, and safe. Consequently, we prefer familiar situations to the unfamiliar and remain close to people, places, and practices we recognize and understand. This means that we'll only wander out into unfamiliar situations when we feel relatively safe *and* need something or are seeking out a new experience.

Six Steps to trust-building:

1. **Start by presenting yourself as a consultant with no skin in the game.** After initiating a new conversation, and we need to posture ourselves as an ally, and not someone who is sitting in judgment. Smile and listen carefully. Additionally, attempt to match body posture, speech pattern, and the tone of voice as the patient's subconscious mind is searching for recognizable patterns in an unfamiliar environment. By matching and mirroring behavior, we can leverage the power of psychosocial *entrainment*.

2. **Maintain an appropriate amount of eye contact.** We project confidence when we maintain eye contact 60 to 70 percent of the time. When a person needs our help, they are simultaneously searching for confidence and caring. So, this is when the adage, "People don't care about how much you know until they know how much you care," comes into play. A caring person who doesn't speak with confidence isn't likely to be considered helpful. On the other hand, when we present as being overly confident, we risk being perceived as self-centered and *less* caring. Hence, the use of a little humility mixed with confidence is likely the most effective approach.

3. **Speak slowly and use a lowered voice.** We sound more confident and caring when we speak slowly and utilize a lower tone of voice. (Bob Barkley was a jovial extrovert. He intentionally modified his communication style to come across as more of an introvert when meeting with patients for the first time). The use of a "slower-lower" tone subconsciously supports the perception that we know what we are talking about, we're not in a hurry, and we sincerely want to help.

4. **Actively listen.** Active listening is the simplest way to demonstrate respect. We don't need to sell ourselves, we need to encourage the patient to share their story. Additionally, we need to curb the impulse to interrupt and inject our thoughts (regardless of how right they might be) too early in a relationship, as it's easily perceived as not being fully present.

5. **Stay in the question**. Ask open-ended questions associated with what was just shared. Mary Osborne, R.D.H., calls this technique "Staying in the Question." If you're genuinely listening, it's an easy thing to do. Once the person supplies more information, a great conversationalist will utilize shared content to ask more open-ended questions until they more fully understand the person's perspective and how they feel about it.

6. **Transition into an advisory role only when you understand the situation from the other person's point of view**. Bob

Barkley famously said, "We must earn the right to care," which is related to the saying, "Nobody values free advice." Why? Because premature advice feels diminishing or irrelevant when it's offered outside of a genuinely caring and helping relationship.

Chapter 22
Empathy and Trust are Related

The word empathy is a popular buzzword in dentistry, but in spite of its popularity, few understand what it means and why it's so important. The confusion is commonly rooted in dictionary definitions such as "the ability to understand and share the feelings of another." Yet, we can't fully understand another person's feelings. In truth, the best we can do is contemplate what a person might be feeling and then project our feelings upon that speculation. That's why Avrom King used to say, "There is no such thing as a second-hand feeling."[64]

Our feelings and our patients' feelings are unique, hence they cannot be fully explained or understood by others. Despite that simple truth, they're both important and valid because what we feel, and how others feel, represent each of our realities. Our brain functions based on thought constructions, that may be reasonably accurate, total fabrications, or something in-between. But in all cases, our thought constructions represent our reality, and the only way to square the accuracy of our thought constructions with the truth is to test them in the real world.

But there's another problem: Our perception of the real world is a thought construction as well. In other words, our brain tests some of our thought constructions against other thought constructions, and when one thought construction is more successful than the other, we call it a "belief." So, you can see that a belief is a temporarily validated thought construction, hence beliefs should always be up for review with regard to accuracy. When we fail to do so on a regular basis, we are at risk of becoming dogmatic.

Why all of this discussion about beliefs, dogma, and empathy? These concepts fully infuse the relationship we have with ourselves and others. *What we think they think influences how we feel, and how we feel influences our behavior.* So, if we enter a new relationship with beliefs about ourselves and others that are rigid and dogmatic, then it's unlikely that we'll discover the whole truth—because we won't be able to understand the situation from the other person's perspective. Yet, it's our patient's perspective that's the main source of motivation to make significant changes—*their* beliefs drive *their* decisions.

How is empathy connected to all of it? Empathy is crucial because it signals we're interested in who they are as a whole person and we don't perceive them as just being another problem to resolve. In other words, empathy signals we think they're significant and their feelings are important to us. When we gift others with our empathy, it allows them to feel safer and accepted, which is a psychological environment which supports their ability to make reassessments and perhaps even change some of their beliefs about dentistry, dentists, and what proper dentistry can do for them. Consequently, we facilitate change in others through empathy, non-judgmental acceptance, and by behaving transparently. Carl Rogers called that "congruence."

Chapter 23
Mary Osborne, R.D.H.

Mary Osborne was practicing in Northern Virginia in 1984, when she was offered a position in Doug Roth's Springfield, Virginia practice.[65] That day, Doug gave Mary a series of cassette tapes titled, *The Nitty Gritty of New Dentistry*. As she listened to the tapes, her reaction was, "Has this guy been living in my head? How can he know so much about how I feel about my professional experiences?" Avrom King's words connected to deep feelings and frustrations that Mary had never explored.

Avrom was a social psychologist who worked closely with Bob Barkley from 1970 to 1977. He was captivated by Bob's thinking and philosophy, and went on to create *Nexus*, a newsletter and a practice consultancy. Doug and Sandy Roth had whole-heartedly committed themselves to the creation of a relationship-based/ health-centered practice, and were one of Avrom's clients.

After listening to Avrom, Mary realized that much of what was being taught to dentists and hygienists wasn't leading to the creation of health, instead, it seemed to encourage the judgment of patients as being either good or bad, compliant or non-compliant. "Avrom talked about patients who would come in and then be told that they were doing a good job. And indeed, that's what happened—they would come in, and we'd tell them they were doing a great job, when in reality all we were doing was acknowledging what we had observed on a given day. In many cases, patients would improve their home care a few days in advance of each visit, and then we'd comment on their thoroughness as it appeared that day, and subsequently we'd misdiagnose their true status."

Doug and Sandy owned a copy of Bob's book *Successful Preventive Dental Practices*, and by reading it, Mary discovered the health-centered philosophy flowing through Avrom King had come from Bob Barkley—someone she knew nothing about. Mary worked with Doug to find ways to apply Bob's knowledge, which was to a large degree focused on understanding how others learn, and then adapting *how they taught* to that new understanding. "Intuitively, I knew that most patients were just trying to do what they were told to do, and that I hadn't been very successful at helping them create long-term preferred outcomes," (because they hadn't yet made the decision to their problems) she said.

Mary and Doug used CoDiscovery as a way to learn more about their patients as they learned more about themselves. Gradually, Mary developed a process she calls, "staying in the question," a communication style that utilizes curiosity to gently probe while interviewing patients.

Doug, Mary, and Sandy were so successful with their person-centered practice model, that other dentists approached them to learn more about how to do it, so they formed an in-house consultancy named *The Roth Group*. Dentists and team members visited their practice to observe how it functioned. The experience included attendance at team meetings and the opportunity to observe how the Roth Team worked through daily challenges and integrated new ideas.

Over time, dentists requested additional onsite help, which led Doug, Mary, and Sandy to form *ProSynergy*, and to base it out of Seattle. Mary went on to form *Mary Osborne Resources* in 1996, where she continues to support dentists and teams in patient care and communication, as well as in the areas of leadership and team building.

Currently, Mary co-facilitates the popular *Leadership and Legacy Retreat* with Joan Unterschuetz and Lee Brady. During the retreat, participants are led through discussions centered around the influence they have on their teams and patients, committing themselves to becoming more effective leaders, better at understanding the needs of their patients, creating healthy workplaces, and how to lead their patients and practices into the future.

When I asked Mary about her passion for the future with regard to advancing the influence Bob Barkley had on her life, she answered:

My most significant learning from Bob Barkley was an understanding of how people learn. Currently, I'm leading a small virtual study club called 'Learning about Learning' that's designed to help people become more skilled at teaching and leading groups so that I can pass on what I learned about Bob Barkley's work.

Chapter 24
Active Listening
At the Core of Empathy and Trust-Building

Carl Rogers wrote, *"We think we listen, but very rarely do we listen with real understanding—true empathy. Yet listening, of this very special kind, is one of the most potent forces for change that I know."*

Active listening plays a central role in all relationship-based/patient-centered practices because it facilitates personal growth and development, which in turn, leads to better decision-making and the advancement of health in more and more sophisticated ways. Active listeners consciously work to fully understand the context of each person's story and the feelings associated with them.

Bob Barkley said when he stopped telling his patients about his practice philosophy and focused his energy on listening, he became a much more effective helper as the shift encouraged each person to develop their own philosophy, and subsequently "...their latent sense of responsibility for their health started to develop."[66] Bob discovered that active listening supported self-initiated learning, which built up each person's confidence in their ability to address complex dental health challenges.

Throughout life, we think of ourselves in particular ways, influenced by our earliest experiences. From there, layers of narratives become a matrix of beliefs stored in our subconscious mind. And it's this matrix — our belief system — that drives our decision-making process, not facts.

Active listening facilitates the reappraisal of a belief system. Reappraisal is a safe process that allows for the exploration of what a person thinks they know and determines if it's still valid. Active listening requires us to think *with* our patients instead of *for* them, hence it's a process that facilitates working *with* others instead of just *on* them.

Active listening is linked to empathy, because both require understanding situations and feelings from another person's perspective. Additionally, active listening involves validation and confirmation once an assessment has been made.

Every communication with a patient has two components:

1. The objective content

2. The feelings associated with the content

Understanding content and the associated emotional valence is important because it helps us to clarify meaning and relevance. In some interview situations, the story's content is less important than the related feelings, as the content may be distorted and the person won't be aware of it. Regardless, the person believes the story is accurate because it has an important meaning to them. Consequently, part of active listening involves discovering the "back story," the narrative in the person's mind that remains unexpressed. For instance, does the person believe they will lose all their teeth regardless of what they do? Do they think losing their teeth is a normal process? Do they believe they are worthy of making a significant investment in themselves? Do they believe, due to previous experiences, that most dental work will fail, and therefore it represents a bad investment? Do they think that most dentists are dishonest because their insurance company communications imply it? Do they believe their problems cannot be successfully resolved, so an episodic, crisis-oriented relationship with dentistry is the way it has to be?

To discover the back story, we must respond to the feeling component of the communication: "You seem upset about what happened. Can you tell me more about it?" "I can see you're anxious. Can you help me understand why you feel that way?" "You seem frustrated—even angry, about what happened to you.

Can you tell me more about it?" By exploring feelings, we discover meaning. Meaning influences a person's motivation to move in one direction or another, so it's important to understand.

How does the person see their experiences in dentistry relative to the arch of their life story, particularly relative to what they're currently experiencing? How do they think their current situation will play out? Is one outcome preferable over another? How much of a priority is it to them to resolve their current challenges? Do they know enough about their current situation to engage in an intelligent discussion and then make good decisions?

Roughly 80% of communication is nonverbal, so our patients' words only convey part of the story. That's why each person must be interviewed, and why we can only learn a little bit from answers given over the phone or written on an intake form. Thus, active listening requires an awareness of all nonverbal and verbal communication. For instance, a patient's hesitant speech pattern reveals something about their feelings. The infection of their voice helps to emphasize a particular aspect of a story. How their eyes move tells us if a person is afraid, ashamed, confident, or evasive. Their eyes might also indicate that the person is too preoccupied with their current problem to discuss anything beyond addressing their chief complaint.

Facial expressions indicate whether or not what the person is saying is congruent with their emotions. In other words, when we pay strategic attention, we can often tell if we are dealing with a fabricated persona or a more authentic person. Other useful nonverbal cues: What is the person doing with their hands? What's their breathing pattern? When we attune ourselves to the presentation of the whole person -physically, verbally, emotionally, and behaviorally, we can more accurately understand content, meaning, motivation, and compatibility.

How we listen conveys a message as well. Does our listening style express: "I am interested in who you are as a person," or "I am just here to gather whatever information is necessary to safely and legally complete this transaction as quickly as possible." Active listening should always imply, "I respect you for who you are. I believe your thoughts and feelings are an integral part of who you are, and you are important to me. I'm confident you can make an important contribution to this relationship. I'm not here to change or judge you; I'm simply trying to figure out the best way to help." Active listening, therefore, demonstrates our purpose through the *quality* of our attention.

Active listening is contagious, which is particularly important when trying to resolve complex situations that require a lot of time, effort, and commitment. The better listener we become, the more likely others will want to carefully listen to us. That's called "earning the right to be heard." Just as anger can beget anger, and deception can beget deception, active listening tends to be reciprocated, particularly when interests and goals are mutually aligned.

Understanding patients on a meaningful level is challenging, so it's helpful to verify what we think we know. That's done by reflecting back what we think we understand: "Let me make sure I understand what you've just told me, you said…." Their response gives us more information about how accurately we have interpreted their situation. A good rule of thumb is to assume that we can never fully understand what a person means until it has been completely confirmed.

Active listening demands a complete setting aside of our biases and assumptions. Hence, active listening requires commitment, practice, and often, a change in our attitude toward others. To become more effective, we must be sincerely interested in our patients and be willing to recognize that a person's feelings, self-narratives, goals, and motivations might differ significantly from our own.

The process also involves an element of risk, as we simultaneously risk the possibility of being changed by the experiences. For instance, when things don't go well for a person under our care, we also feel frustrated, disappointed, or even feel their pain. That can be transformative in both positive and negative ways, hence, it takes a certain amount of courage to pursue deeper understanding and to help others in profound ways. Along the way, we'll hear expressions like, "I hate dentists," or "I would rather have a baby…," and sometimes it's hard to hear that without becoming defensive or cynical. It can, therefore, require some personal work to get ourselves to a place where we can hear these expressions as cries for help.

Questions: How often do you use active listening in your practice? How can you allow active listening to occur more frequently? How do you think your practice will change if you strategically use active listening as your primary form of communication?

Chapter 25
Gary Takacs

Born in Cleveland, Ohio to Hungarian immigrants, Gary spent his junior and high school years in San Diego, California.[67] He met David Hornbrook the summer before his freshman year, and they became surfing buddies and lifelong friends. Gary went on to graduate from the University of Oregon with a degree in History and an eye on law school—not for the purpose of practicing law, but to use as part of his skillset as a consultant.

Gary never made it to law school, due to working closely with Rick Mercer at his consultancy focused on helping dental practices. After a few years, Gary decided to strike out on his own, but another opportunity suddenly presented itself that he couldn't refuse. "The ink on my new business cards was hardly dry, when I got a call out of the blue from Omer Reed,"[68] he said. Burt Press had recommended Gary as a possible candidate to join Omer in his new organization called *Pentegra*. Omer was so impressed by Burt's recommendation, that he decided to fly Gary down to discuss a possible future together.

Gary joined Omer and was soon exposed to the work of Bob Barkley for the very first time. Omer had a library full of books, pamphlets, and other material he used for writing and teaching purposes, with much of it related to Bob Barkley. Omer had integrated Bob's concept of an oral health learning center focused on disease prevention, oral health skills development, and dietary counseling.

Omer Reed's relationship with Bob Barkley dated back to the mid-1960's when they were both prominent speakers on the national lecture circuit. Consequently, Omer Reed frequently mentioned Bob's influence on his own work:

Perhaps the key to me was the work of the great, late Robert Barkley who, in an unprecedented fashion, provided us with the concept of CoDiscovery in the hearts, minds, values, and mouths of those who came to us for care. Hot on the heels of that phenomenon was his Co-Treatment Planning, which began at the pace of the person coming to us for care. We, as a service team, provided patients with what they valued the most – health!

In addition, Omer frequently talked about how dentists need to find a way to free themselves from the codependency bonds created by the insurance industry:

It's astoundingly true that people pay gladly for that which they value, so that myths in dentistry, such as cash sensitivity, piecework sensitivity, and time sensitivity, fade into total insignificance for those who conceive as did Barkley. So, without question, Barkley's work with Dr. Pankey in regard to the "sliding fee schedule" is unperceived by most people in dentistry, and the co-development of a fee that's fair grows only in the practices of a few private care-oriented dental crews who understand how that works.

Gary Takacs went on to consult with over 2000 dentists and help many practices transition out of insurance dependency, through the integration of CoDiscovery, CoDiagnosis, and Co-Treatment Planning in combination with many other strategic management principles. Additionally, he co-founded a dental practice called *Life Smiles* in Phoenix, Arizona with Paul Nielson and Tim Schmidt. Gary is a visiting faculty member of the Pankey Institute and a frequent co-presenter at Bob Barkley Study Club workshops.

The implication of this euphemism is that the medical care system, collectively speaking, and physicians individually, are the ultimate source of everyone's health. But the truth is that health can no more be imparted by one person to another than wisdom, courage, integrity, or any other desirable human quality can be.

The medical community's reinforcement of this myth, along with politicians' advancing of it, has created a deep sense of psychological dependence in the public's mind with doctors. And as a result, our society has become more "medicalized," while healthcare has been progressively expropriated by the vast, medical-industrial complex, to mostly shareholders' gain.

~Avrom E. King,

The Nitty Gritty of New Dentistry

Chapter 26
Why Is the New Patient Here?

When we meet a new patient for the very first time, it's critically important to know *why* they've come, meaning—what are their concerns, motivating factors, priorities, and values relative to dental health and treatment? If we fail to discern who this person truly is, and why they're sitting in front of us, then we are only able function from a place of superficial analysis and assumptions—both of which are incomplete orientations that can easily lead to misunderstandings.

Generally speaking, a person enters our office for one of four reasons:

1. They have an acute problem that needs immediate resolution and it's simple to resolve.

2. They have a problem that requires a complicated solution, they have no concept of the complexity of their problem, and they are primarily focused on their discomfort, disability, embarrassment, or dysfunction.

3. They have no perceived needs (although they may have many actual needs). A third party, such as a dental insurance carrier, has prompted them to seek out services.

4. They have a goal in mind that's based upon a desire to improve their health, comfort, or appearance.

Each reason has a different motivating factor that involves a different decision-making process. When we understand their reason, we can facilitate better decisions that move the relationship closer to a "win-win" orientation. If we fail to understand the person's motivations, we're functionally chasing a black cat around a dark room. And that's why Dr. Pankey famously said, "Know Your Patient;" he wasn't referring to just "knowing" their dental needs. He was referring to knowing each person on a more holistic level: who they are physically, emotionally, temperament-wise, and motivation-wise. And what is their financial capacity to manage the cost of a challenging rehabilitative project?

Bob Barkley liked to call a person's chief complaint their "present preoccupation," because it was usually an incomplete understanding. For example, a person might say, "My jaw joint hurts every time I eat, and it's driving me crazy. I can't enjoy a meal with my family," or "Can you help me? I don't know what's wrong, something doesn't feel right." Many dentists immediately jump into a comprehensive examination, create a list of everything that appears to need correction or attention, and then try to gain approval to proceed. This is not to say we shouldn't be doing comprehensive examinations; rather, we're often *not being comprehensive enough* because we've skipped past taking the time to truly understand who the person is, why they're present, how they feel about their situation, and their commitment level.

Any good salesperson worth their salt, selling a complex product or service, knows they must see the problem – the reason the client called the company in the first place, from the perspective of the client, *before* they propose a solution to the perceived needs. Otherwise, they won't be selling much of anything to anyone because they are functionally *cold calling.*

When Avrom King was a young business consultant, he proposed a complex solution to a Board of Directors struggling with a complex problem after only knowing them for a few hours. Immediately after the meeting, Avrom's boss pulled him aside and said, "If you ever do that again you're fired!" Avrom was confused and asked, "Was my analysis wrong?" His boss responded, "Probably not." Avrom then asked, "Was my solution wrong?" and his boss answered, "Perhaps incomplete but probably not wrong." "Then why are you angry?" asked Avrom. His boss's answer was illuminating:

You demeaned the client. You took their dignity. These are bright men, and they have spent their lives in business. You're a punk kid with no experience, and after just two hours, you're telling them how to do their jobs. I'm pretty sure they can stand up to your audacity, but King, I fear for your soul if you think the consulting business is about defining problems and creating solutions.[69]

Reflect on this story for a moment, as we all make similar mistakes, and when our ideas aren't immediately accepted, we blame the person for having a "low dental IQ" or "not valuing proper dentistry." I'd like to suggest that many of those assumptions are more rationalizations than reality; the main problem might be that we haven't yet earned the right to be heard.

Do the best you can until you know better, then when you know better—do better.

~Maya Angelou

All God's Children Need Traveling Shoes, Vintage Press (1962)

Chapter 27
William C. Strupp, Jr., DDS

Most dentists are familiar with the impressive clinical work of Bill Strupp, and his long career as a top speaker.[70] However, few people are aware of Bill's connection to Bob Barkley. Bill is a native of Greenville, Florida. His grandfather was a Florida State Senator and a highly regarded merchant. Bill's father was an aviator who trained pilots during World War II.

Bill graduated early at the top of his high school class in Greenville with valedictorian honors, despite dyslexia and an inability to read proficiently until the 6th grade. Bill considered becoming an engineer after Clemson University invited him to a two-week summer camp, but his career path shifted toward dentistry after his childhood orthodontist shared the financial and lifestyle benefits of the field.

Bill attended Oxford College of Emory University at age 17, graduating with a BA degree and the highest score in organic chemistry. He then studied dentistry at Emory and graduated in 1969. Bill said that his personality and dental school's *"I said so,"* culture didn't mesh well, and he subsequently ended up in the bottom third of his graduating class. *"Dental school was a bust for me – I was constantly in trouble,"* he said.

The Vietnam War peaked in 1969, so instead of risking the draft and losing control of his future, Bill joined the Air Force and was stationed at the Richards-Gebaur AFB near Kansas City. *"I had the worst officer efficiency rating of anyone on the base,"* Bill said with a laugh. (Officer efficiency ratings were based upon how well a person followed protocol regarding proper wearing of the uniform, saluting, and other military traditions.) In spite of his reluctance to conform to military ways, Bill was the most productive dentist on the base and was subsequently assigned Preventive Dentistry Officer duties.

As the Preventive Dental Officer, Bill was responsible for creating written oral health protocols for all base personnel. That was when he came in contact with Bob Barkley's work. *"The military and I weren't a good fit,"* he said, *"but it was good for me to see what socialized dentistry would look like; everything was mediocre."*

Bill would go on to set up a solo practice in Clearwater, Florida, "after watching everyone *doing 4-pin amalgams and cementing their crowns in pools of blood, I knew there had to be a better way,"* he said. Bill took courses from Niles Guichet, L.D. Pankey and Peter Dawson, among others, "There are so many things you can learn and teach yourself if you're just willing to do the work. When I was 25 years old, I took three philosophy courses from L.D. Pankey, and I finally got myself to the point where I couldn't work on a patient other than in a comprehensive way, and with lifelong goals in mind."

In 1974, Bill put together his own presentation, which he now attributes most of his professional growth, as he had to not only understand the material on a deep level, but he also had to prepare himself for all potential questions.

On Saturday, August 13, 1977, Bill attended a meeting of The Sarasota County Dental Association, where Bob Barkley was speaking on philosophy and disease prevention. At that point, Bill had heard Bob speak at least ten times and had integrated much of Bob's philosophy into his practice. When Bob saw Bill, he asked, "What are you doing here? You could be teaching this course at this point!" to which Bill responded, "Maybe I'll hear it differently this time!" — and they laughed.

That day, part of Bob's presentation was about future-focusing, followed by an exercise requiring each person to write down their obituary as it would appear in the local dental newsletter. Bill asked Bob, "What will you write down today?" and Bob answered,

"I don't know, but whatever it is, I don't want to be called "Pied Piper of Plaque!" and again they laughed.

Later that night, Bob's chartered plane out of Chicago crashed in a field northeast of Macomb near Bushnell; Bob had successfully made it from Tampa to Chicago and was on the last leg of his trip home. The plane carried only three passengers: Bob, the pilot, and the co-pilot. Combined, they had hundreds of hours of flight experience, yet they were unable to save the plane. Witnesses on the ground stated that the cabin was full of black smoke.

When I asked Bill to share the most important things that he learned from Bob Barkley, he quickly answered:

People have more value for their teeth after they get their disease under control. Once I understood that, I never had to hard-sell dentistry because you can't expect people to do something that they don't understand or value. And they certainly don't want to do it when they don't trust you. People come in who know about us, but they know next to nothing of us; so, they're almost always full of misconceptions. It's our job to help them learn our preventive philosophy and to get them to want the dentistry they need — dentistry that will last them a lifetime.

Chapter 28
Perception and Behavior are Driven by Meaning

I t's easy to feel overwhelmed by the constant exposure to a flow of information that's inside and outside of our control. Our brain is designed for one primary purpose: self-preservation, and not for complete understanding, prioritizing, accurately remembering, and appropriately responding to everything that's sensed. And when tasked with too much responsibility, the brain will simplify decision-making down to instincts instead of using objective analysis. In other words, situations that cause confusion, feel threatening, or contain too many unknowns, trigger the limbic system to take control and drive the behavior pattern— often in unbalanced and unproductive ways.

Our brain also has a natural tendency toward *conservatism*—an inherent desire to maintain the status quo even when our behavior creates an unsatisfactory outcome. Fear, for instance, often causes withdrawal and the seeking out of familiar comforts. Although this instinctive strategy feels safe, it shuts down creative problem-solving. Fight, flight, or freeze are supposed to be quick responses, yet many people live a lifestyle that's predominantly fear-driven or avoidance-of-fear driven.

The good news is that fear and anxiety can be overcome through the development of a profoundly purposeful plan driven by our *why*. A deeply intentional plan shifts our brain away from our anxious limbic system and up to a more thoughtful and productive prefrontal cortex. When our plan includes a clear vision of our preferred future, our brain will start to function *as if* that perspective is already true and will start to search for ways to support it. Maxwell Maltz, M.D., wrote an entire book on this amazing phenomenon titled *Psycho-Cybernetics*.[71]

From a neuroscience perspective, what captures our attention the most is personal meaning—something that occurs before we even realize it. Our brain reacts to information and situations relative to its understanding of what it thinks it means—and not based upon what's true or what it actually represents. (Recall Tom's comment earlier in Chapter 17: "The world is full of information, but the challenge is that most of that information has yet to be translated into practical knowledge.")

The legendary German philosopher Martin Heidegger was convinced that meaning drives behavior.[72] He hypothesized that we each have a unique perspective of the world that's based upon our unique interpretation of experiences. Hence, we perceive the world through a lens tinted by unique meanings.

That type of thinking feels foreign today, as our culture has largely shifted its perspective toward materialistic and secular philosophies. Deeply materialistic and secular philosophies lack meaning and generate a pervasive sense of nihilism, which can lead to anxiety and freezing, failing to act decisively at critically important times.

If we deeply explore anything physical, it's initially perceived as shapes that can be broken down into smaller and smaller subunits: cells, atoms, electrons, which can be further broken down to energy behaving in predictable patterns. Why are things this way? How did all of this happen? The answers to these questions can only be found in disciplines of philosophy and religion—and not objective science.

How is any of this relevant to the practice of dentistry? Because everything I've shared with you holds true for our patients as well. Our patients must find their *why* if we want them to make better health-centered decisions, as well as find the motivation to carry them out. Our patients must understand the *meaning* of our proposed treatment strategy within the context of what's most relevant and important to them. So, our process of recommending solutions must involve much more than simply pointing out physical or functional deficits and negotiating a payment plan.

Stay away from those people who try to disparage your ambitions. Small minds will always do that, but great minds will give you a feeling that you can become great too.

~ Mark Twain (Harnsberger, C.

Mark Twain at Your Fingertips, Dover Publications, 1946

Chapter 29
People Can Change, But We Can't Change Them

In one Seth Godin's recent blog posts, he wrote:

If you open a roadside motel, expect that tired and demanding budget travelers will arrive. If you run a fancy restaurant, don't be surprised if people angle, cajole, and lie to get a 'better' table. If you hustle to get market share, you'll probably end up with customers who insist on ever more hustle and trickery to stay with you. If you decide to become a coach, realize that most of your prospects will be people who don't think they need a coach. (Because the people who want and need a coach already have one). If you attract new freelance business by being the cheapest, I'm betting that your customers will give you a hard time about your rates. If you're a mental health professional, expect that the people you encounter will have issues with their mental health. Sometimes, things work the way they are supposed to, even if it's not what we might want in the moment.

As dentists, the same holds true. The vast majority of our patients focus on what they think someone else should have to pay rather than on their health or the long-term strategies they need to deploy to remain healthy. Why? Because they've been trained to think in that way by dental insurance companies, and by dentists who take dental insurance as a proxy form of currency. In the world of heuristics, that tendency is called "scarcity bias." We have a natural tendency to conserve resources, particularly when we don't have enough information to know when to trade our limited resources for something we think is more valuable. (Note that I *am not* saying, "when we should trade someone else's resources for something we've been told that we need.")

How much does a person value their health? The answer to that question is what Bob Barkley referred to as "their philosophy." Therefore, it's important to understand our patient's philosophy and how much it has been influenced by scarcity bias. Bob Barkley, at one point, told all of his patients about *his* philosophy at the first appointment. He even had a detailed brochure that explained why they would be doing things his way. But his logic-driven approach turned out to be a bust.

Bob, through his work with Nate Kohn Jr., PhD., eventually came to a new realization:

Nate knew that with no course in philosophy development and virtually no behavioral training, I was sliding along in previously laid out paths. He helped me to see that while I was no longer creating edentulous mouths, I probably was still performing countless other obsolete tasks. We discovered that my preventive work, which at that time was just beginning, called for vastly different patient-management techniques—techniques that forced me out of well-worn paths. Together we resolved that these things would no longer stymie my growth...As an educational psychologist, Nate was appalled at attempts being made by dentists to educate people...He said that, unfortunately, through their psychological naivety, dentists blame the patients for not wanting the work they propose done, instead of recognizing that the problem is their own inability to establish an effective working relationship with their patients.[73]

As a result, Bob flipped his examination process upside down: instead of attempting to sell *his* philosophy to those who had a minimal capacity to understand its relevance, he tried to understand what was most important to each person. From there, he strategically contrasted where they were health-wise, against where they thought they were, including how things were trending. That was a connection that most people could not make on their own—it required facilitation. In other words, Bob helped the person verbalize what was most important to them and then explored what it would mean to them if they weren't able to sustain it.

A good writer possesses not only his own spirit, but also the spirit of his friends.

~Friedrich Nietzsche

Chapter 30
Lynn D. Carlisle, D.D.S.

Lynn Carlisle practiced dentistry in Fort Collins, Colorado beginning in 1968. Like many dentists, Lynn was overwhelmed by the many things he needed to learn to become successful. Consequently, Lynn pursued personal and professional development to a high degree. Along the way, he worked with Omer Reed, Carl Rogers, Arthur Combs, Wilson Southam, Doug Young, Mike Schuster, Avrom King, and studied at The Pankey Institute. Additionally, Lynn was a voracious reader and subsequently integrated the work of Toffler, Drucker, Combs, Maslow, Pankey, Barkley, Kohn, in addition to many others.[74]

Lynn used his deep understanding and writing skills to create a part memoir, part guidebook titled *In a Spirit of Caring* in 1994,[75] which was very well-received within the person-centered / health-centered community. The legendary Henry Tanner, one of Lynn's instructors at The Pankey Institute, said, "I read your book three times, it is the best book on the subject I have ever read, and the best book I have read this year." Doug and Marylyn Young said of it, "Lynn's sensitive, insightful portrait of self-discovery is an essential resource for every member of the health care team."

In a Spirit of Caring is still available on Kindle™ and used print copies can be found. I highly recommend reading Lynn's book for the purpose of reminding yourself that self-development is never a straight-line, upward process. It requires many side journeys and disappointments along the road toward mastery. To quote Jordan Peterson, "If you aren't willing to first be a fool, you can never be a master."

Lynn's book was instrumental in my journey, and our friendship was primarily responsible for my ability to write *this* book. My relationship with Lynn also led me to take a *New Patient*

Experience course from Bob Frazer,[76] someone who was also significantly influenced by Bob Barkley's work.

I'd like to share a few quotes from *In a Spirit of Caring* for the purpose of prompting you to download the book on Kindle™ or to track down a used copy:

Like lost souls, dentists have lost touch with the human dimensions of dentistry, especially the caring doctor-patient relationship built upon a reciprocal compassion, caring and respect between doctor and patient.

The public perception of dentists and physicians is that they have been seduced by technology, money and specialization. They have little concern for patients and their questions, concerns, wants and needs.

Physicians and dentists are feeling a loss of control of their professional lives as third parties attempt to manage health care decisions with interventions and regulations that endanger a caring doctor-patient relationship.

Besides dental treatment and prevention of dental disease, dentistry is in the behavior change and lifestyle business.

Most patients that seek dental treatment are physically healthy. They can make sentient decisions with their full faculties. This provides the dental team with opportunities to build long-term relationships.

The finest dentistry is discretionary.

Caring asks the dentist to be fully present and to be fully authentic and congruent during interactions with patients.

If we withhold our humanness, we hide the very ingredients that give meaning and direction to our own lives and impair our ability to help our clients grow and heal.

There was a frantic search for the magic ingredient to make my practice life fulfilling. I was searching outside myself for the magic solution. There was persistence in my search. As I struggled, I blamed others for my shortcomings...As long as I continued to look outside, success eluded me. When I looked inside, I found the path to fulfillment.

Note: Bob Frazer went through a similar disenchantment period while in dental school, during which time he had the serendipitous opportunity to hear Bob Barkley speak. About that experience, Bob said:

First, in my heart and mind, he was the man most responsible for me becoming a dentist and the teacher I am within our great profession today...I sat toward the back of the room as I listened to this passionate man speak of his similar high-fear, low-trust dental school experience...That's how it felt!... Although everything he said made the greatest sense to me, it wasn't until he said, "You who are training to be dentists will have a greater opportunity to really help people (more) than any medical profession, because in the absence of pain, bleeding, and swelling, people don't need to come to you, but they will anyway. That was when my epiphany occurred.

Chapter 31
Understanding the Work of Carl Jung

Psychology is the scientific study of the mind and behavior, including the study of conscious and unconscious phenomena, feelings, and thoughts. Understanding psychology is essential to person-centered dentistry because it helps us to better understand ourselves, our team, and our patients. It also helps us address our daily challenges more easily by opening the door to more holistic perspectives.

In our high-obligation, high-expectation, high-stress world, it's easy to feel overwhelmed and directionless as we run from one commitment, obligation, or crisis to the next. When we develop the ability to step back and establish a wiser perspective, we discover that life is rich in meaning, potentialities, purpose, connection, and joy—our point of view shifts from frantic to acknowledging that life is filled with experiences that we can choose to participate in—or not.

Carl Gustav Jung (1875–1961) was a Swiss-born psychologist who initially studied under Sigmund Freud and went on to develop his own theories. To explain the difference between Jung and Freud in the simplest terms: Jung saw people as full of potential and possibilities, whereas Freud's perspective was more medicalized and focused on what was wrong.[77]

As a result, Jung became a thought leader in the modern psychotherapy movement, a facilitated process of self-exploration for the purpose of creating opportunities for positive change. Facilitated self-reflection helps uncover who a person truly is beneath all of their subconscious habits, behavior patterns, thoughts, and worldview. Most people spend very little time studying themselves because they're too busy, too distracted, too upset, or too tired. Yet, doing so with a sense of purpose can significantly impact the quality, of a person's life.

Jung is best known for his theory of the psyche as being a multifaceted mental system formed from a combination of unconscious thoughts driven by unexamined beliefs (the shadow), our conscious self and associated thoughts, and meta-narratives shared by everyone—archetypes. He also coined the term "synchronicity" to describe coincidences that appear meaningful in hindsight. In other words, when we align our behavior, beliefs, and agendas with our purpose, we start to see that many "coincidences" have a spiritual component to them.

Jung believed that each person has a "shadow side" (unexamined memories and associated beliefs) hidden from view but capable of being reexamined and reinterpreted in helpful ways. Jung believed that the way we interpret life events, consciously and unconsciously, plays a significant role in how our personality develops over time. "It all depends on how we look at things and not how they are in themselves," Jung said. By paying attention to how we respond to events, we can better understand ourselves and the motivations behind various behavior patterns. When we understand these concepts, we are able to see their relevance when applied to the practice of dentistry:

> Most people don't know where they are dental-health-wise, don't know how they got there, don't know where they are headed health-wise, and therefore are largely unable to make good long-term decisions regarding their dental health.

> Most dentists don't know themselves, don't understand how the mind works, and resort to positional power or manipulation to cause their patients to take action, which in turn creates codependency relationships they resent.

Developing ourselves and our patients is challenging, because it takes time, but it's also where "happiness" resides.

Know all the theories. Master all of the techniques. But as you touch a human soul, be just another human soul.

~ Carl Jung, PhD

Chapter 32
What Is "Authenticity" and Why Is it Important?

We're often told to "be authentic," but what does the really mean? Avrom King said, "The Authentic Self is our most pure, least distorted sense of ourselves." In Jungian terms, it refers to a well-integrated ego, wherein a person has done lot of self-work to understand the subconscious drivers behind their negative behavior, and subsequently have made numerous positive changes.

Another way to conceptualize authenticity is when our persona – our public "mask" is in alignment with how we think and feel. Thus, when we're behaving in a more authentic fashion, our public mask is minimized—we're more *transparent*, and as a result, others can more easily see who we are and respond appropriately to our intentions.

It's unrealistic to think that someday we'll reach a point when we'll never need to function behind a social mask. For example, when we initiate a new relationship, we'll use a social mask: we'll stand up straight, smile, and look the person in the eye. Typically, in response, they'll do something similar, and positive feelings will start to flow in both directions. We commonly call these experiences "good rapport," but good rapport is largely superficial and has minimal influence on significant learning and the change dynamic.

That's *why* authenticity / transparency are important; they provide the pathway through which positive change is most predictably facilitated—because authenticity begets authenticity. When one person opens up and honestly shares their feelings in a nonjudgmental fashion, it leads to reciprocation, which leads to greater awareness, a change in perspective, beliefs, behavior, and outcomes.

If all of this authenticity stuff sounds easy—it's not. It's quite challenging to be fully open and honest at the right times. Why? Because authenticity and transparency leave us vulnerable to judgment and rejection, consequently, we're fully transparent only on a selective basis—only with our closest friends and allies. So, don't be confused, I'm not suggesting that we need to function in a fully transparent fashion all of the time. Rather, I'm suggesting that we should be authentic and fully transparent with *some* people, *some* of the time, for the purpose of personal growth, development, and positive change. At other times, we need to be *strategic*, and try to set the stage for more opportunities for authenticity to evolve.

Chapter 33
Abundance, Scarcity, Boundary, and Healthy Relationships

The concepts of abundance, perspective, and psychological boundary are *primary* with regard to how our brain functions. They also represent the irreducible building blocks upon which our personality develops over time. Primary building blocks are created during childhood and directly influence our worldview. Our worldview subsequently has a significant influence on our capacity to learn, grow, and optimally function.

When a person's primary building blocks are well-designed and strong, the person emerges from adolescence with a relatively clear and undistorted sense of self. That clarity yields a confident, kind, curious, humble, loving, growth-oriented personality—a person with a high level of self-regard. When the primary building blocks are poorly constructed, the personality is negatively influenced by confusion and uncertainty, which leads to fear, stress, and a desire to reduce stress by attempting to control the environment. The drive to control the environment includes the desire to control the self and others (with some common symptoms being anorexia, addictions, neurosis, psychosis, etc.). It also includes attempts to control emotional responses, which the insecure person experiences as uncomfortable and unruly.

You're likely able to identify with one or another of these perspectives—secure or insecure, "open" or "closed"—as well as notice the pattern in others. A person with underdeveloped primary building blocks is commonly perceived as being interpersonally cold and insensitive (this can also be hidden behind a false charisma -an unauthentic and learned behavior pattern designed to manipulate). On the other hand, individuals with solid primary building blocks have warm, sensitive personalities and are quickly responsive to the needs of others. They tend to worry less, learn more easily, move past adversity with more poise, and accept themselves for who they truly are.

Abundance

When we talk about the concept of abundance, we're referring to a mindset associated with a generally positive perspective of how the world works. The perspective can be stated as: *My world is generally safe and predictable, as it usually provides me with what I need to be happy and successful at what I feel is most important in my life.*

As a consequence, this type of person is outwardly joyful and generally grateful. The abundant worldview is organic in the sense that it's the way we're all designed to live and function. Our innate tendency toward an abundance perspective was either supported or undermined by how we were raised, and by what we experienced, particularly during the first five years of our life. Thus, the quality of the *nurture* we received, plus our *life experiences,* led us toward developing either an abundance or a scarcity perspective.

Reflection: If you entered dental school with a scarcity mindset, it is likely that you had a very difficult time adapting to all of the critiques and criticism, as you were more prone to taking the feedback personally. Dental team members are affected by this psychological phenomenon as well. That's why we want to hire people with an abundance perspective, particularly for the most public-facing positions. Finally, our patients will present with one or the other of these perspectives. People with a scarcity-mindset tend to be cynical and slow to learn; hence, we will need to move more slowly with them, or choose not to engage them at all if they are unable to establish a successful, collaborative relationship with our practice.

When children are nurtured and supported by "good enough" parenting and protection (and by that, I mean no parenting is/was perfectly executed), the child emerges with a rather clear sense of who they are (which includes a full range of emotional responses they are capable of appropriately processing and expressing)—which leads into the development of an adult who generally feels safe, included, joyful, curious, and creative.

Scarcity

Now, let's look at the other side of the very same coin: *The Scarcity Mindset.* The scarcity mindset is a learned set of thought patterns that override a person's inherent abundance perspective. The scarcity mindset represents a belief system that's supported by a perspective that assumes the best way to get ahead in life is to accumulate and hoard as much as possible, because there can never be enough of anything to feel safe and secure. Scarcity, therefore, is a fear-driven thought pattern fixated on measuring, monitoring, manipulating, and maintaining. Instead of a cool, calm, and collected emotional profile, the scarcity mindset is driven by a deep sense of inadequacy, anxiety, and loss-aversion. Avrom King described the tendency as, "Control is manifested by a deep need to protect the self rather than the desire to enjoy and to serve."

The cynical scarcity posture feeds upon itself to create a self-fulfilling prophecy: negative expectations are realized more often because every challenge is approached with a negative attitude. That's why a person with a scarcity mindset is functionally un-creative—they spend most of their time making sure that no one trespasses on their beliefs and feelings. It's a pattern commonly seen in bullies—people who are at their core emotionally insecure, dominating, and manipulative.

People who develop a scarcity perspective tend to be ineffective at creating and managing intimate (authentic) relationships. My use of the word "intimate" here is related to a person's ability to freely communicate feelings, perspectives, and intentions. Emotionally intimate (authentic) relationships are at the center of every successful relationship-based/health-centered practice. And that's because it's only through emotional intimacy that personal truths and values-driven desires are revealed, safely discussed, and appropriately addressed.

Boundary

The concept of interpersonal boundaries is straightforward: we can't establish a boundary around something that isn't defined. A clear personal boundary begins with understanding who we are, what we believe, what we are willing to defend, and how much we are willing to suffer to advance our beliefs and priorities.

Our psychological boundary represents our defense, growth, and sustenance system. Consequently, we can't maintain, defend, or advance much of anything without a functional boundary.

Psychologically speaking, our boundary represents the outer perimeter of our true self—the place where our responsibility ends. Simultaneously, it marks where others' responsibilities begin.

A fully functional boundary acts like a regulator with a series of controllable gates. The gates regulate what's allowed inside (and therefore what influences the true self) and what is kept outside. Because boundaries are managed differently by different people, everyone's personality is different. Gate functionality can fall on a spectrum of "too closed" on the one end and "too open" on the other. When boundary gates are too closed, a person blocks out intimacy, and when they do, they block out the useful emotional information that comes along with it. As a result, a person with over-controlled boundaries tends to make decisions based upon inaccurate assumptions, which then lead into more frustrations because their assumptions are frequently proven wrong over time.[78]

On the other end of the spectrum, when a boundary system is too porous, it disrupts the person's capacity to recognize and honor their own needs and wants. Hence, interpersonal boundaries that are too porous throw a person's life out of balance as their needs are repeatedly left unaddressed—a scenario that creates so much internal confusion, that the person begins to look outside of themselves for confirmation of their self-worth.

Know Yourself

All of these concepts relate back to why Dr. Pankey taught: "Know Yourself," which is a life-long process of answering the following questions:

1. Do I have a scarcity or abundance mindset?

2. Do I have a psychological boundary that serves me and my patients well?

3. If I take into consideration my current mindset and boundary, are there improvements I can make that will catalyze growth and allow me to help myself and others in more significant ways?

4. Am I able to love my patients enough that they're able to sense it, and subsequently feel safe in following my well-intended leadership—hence *quid pro quo* is my most powerful practice development tool?

Chapter 34
Gary DeWood, DDS, MS

Gary DeWood is a 1980 graduate of Case Western School of Dentistry.[79] Gary and Cheryl Davis were dental school classmates who married after their second year. The primary reason according to Gary: "because it saved money on book purchases." They must still be saving money on books since they're still together 45 years later! After completion of their GPR residencies, they joined forces to launch a practice in Pemberville, Ohio, population 1200. Pemberville is located about 50 miles southeast of Toledo in an area surrounded by family farms. "I learned a lot about the value of relationships living in that community; it was a great place to raise kids," Gary said.

Gary and Cheryl used a new patient survey over a period of several years to discover that 94 out of 100 of adult new patients entering the practice believed that they were in *Excellent* or *Good* dental health, and they felt that they didn't need any significant amount of dentistry to reach their goal of lifetime dental health. Gary saw their situation differently and took the large gap between what people tended to believe and the reality of their health status as a challenge. Consequently, he committed himself to finding ways to "help people see that what they had (health-wise) could get in the way of what they wanted—even when they believed they were healthy."

Taking a first step in the direction of that pursuit, Gary attended *The Pankey Institute* and started to learn about "behavioral dentistry." Rich Green became his mentor and a lifelong friend. Soon Gary was reading books, watching videotapes, and recording his conversations with his patients. One of those videotapes was of Bob Barkley conducting a new patient examination, and one of the books was Barkley's *Successful Preventive Dental Practices*. In a 2014 presentation to the American Academy of Fixed Prosthodontics, Gary said:

My goal initially was to be the best I could possibly be at understanding and applying the science and applying the logic...I worked hard to get my patients to see the logic, and thought that if I mastered the science, it would lead to 'yes'... and then if they weren't able to see the logic, I thought I needed a bigger screen, or a better tool...People often come to us with their mouth open and their ears closed...Why don't people act? It's not so much about them <u>not</u> knowing, it's more about owning; it's about asking, it's about emotion, and it's about experiencing.

In the 90s, Gary and Cheryl brought Mary Osborne into their practice to gain even more exposure to the concepts of CoDiscovery and CoDiagnosis. Mary helped them learn how to become more effective educators and leaders, and as a result, the restorative and prosthodontic side of their practice took off.

In 2002, Cheryl entered an orthodontic residency at the University of Tennessee and, upon graduation, was asked to take over as Clinic Director for Graduate Orthodontics. Simultaneously, Gary transitioned the Pemberville practice over to a new owner while finishing his master's degree in Biomedical Sciences at the University of Toledo College of Medicine. Next, he took over as the Clinical Director at The Pankey Institute. During that period, Gary lived with Rich Green part of the time, which allowed him the opportunity to further discuss Rich Green's experiences with Bob Barkley and L.D. Pankey.

In 2008, Gary left the Pankey Institute to help transform Frank Spear's *Seattle Institute* into *Spear Education.*® Within six months of his arrival, the organization was moved to Scottsdale, Arizona, into a bigger facility where Gary assumed the role of Executive Vice President, developed strategic plans, curriculum, and taught courses. Cheryl joined him in Phoenix in 2009 to establish an orthodontic practice in Phoenix as well as Bellevue, Washington.

Gary's message to the profession:

Patients don't take action because they haven't yet become emotionally involved in their condition. We need to change how patients think about dental health and how they experience dentistry. We need to talk less about treatment plans until the patient asks us to solve an issue they have with them. We need to help them hear, so they can ask. We need to become students of people with the same enthusiasm and energy that we became students of dentistry.

I didn't always know what I was feeling because I had been programmed to suppress my emotions while spending most of my time worrying about how others felt, what they wanted, what they needed, and what they thought about me. Today, I'm much more in touch with my own thoughts, my feelings, my aspirations, and my goals.

~Lisa Roman

The Road Back to Me

Chapter 35
Understanding Co-Dependency

Co-dependency[80] represents a cluster of behaviors that lead toward unhealthy relationships. In a dental practice, the level of co-dependency present within a relationship can vary from one patient to the next. To better visualize this concept, imagine co-dependency on a continuum, with a minimal amount present on the right side under the word *caregiving* and a maximal level of co-dependency on the left under the word *caretaking*:

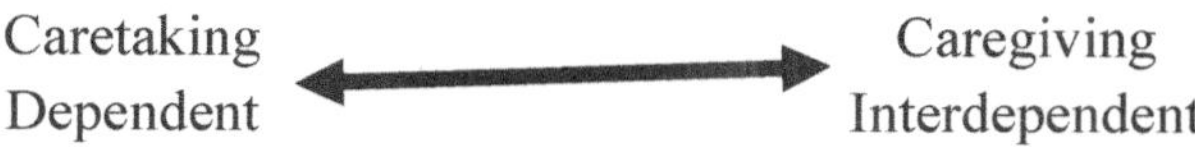

When we're primarily in caretaking mode, we are functioning in a dependency relationship wherein both members of the relationship need each other. That mutual need is the main driver behind the desire to maintain the status quo. On the other hand, when we're primarily in a caregiving mode, we're mainly in an interdependent, volitional, and expansive relationship. So, dependency relationships focus on sustaining the status quo, while interdependent relationships are dynamic and tend to be growth-oriented.

What's another difference? Intention.

In reality, we often find ourselves acting as both caretaker and caregiver in our more intimate relationships, with one role taking precedence over the other at different times.

For example, we all begin as infants who need 100% caretaking and evolve into young adults who require more caregiving. From there, we transition into an elderly stage wherein we again need more and more caretaking. Therefore, the cycle of life is a cycle of dependency evolving into more and more interdependency and then back again.

Now, let's relate these concepts to a relationship-based/health-centered practice, which aims to reduce excessive caretaking. Too much patient dependency on caretaking stifles learning and growth; hence, too much caretaking stifles progression toward higher levels of interdependence. If too many of our patients require caretaking, then our practice's growth and development can easily become impaired.

How can we know how a particular relationship is trending?

Hints:

Caretaking tends to be stressful, whereas caregiving tends to be energizing.

Caretaking tends to violate interpersonal boundaries, whereas caregiving tends to respect them. Consequently, in the former, we often feel like we are giving too much of ourselves to sustain the relationship. In contrast, the process of caregiving feels like we are gaining as much or more from the relationship than we are giving.

Caretaking tends to attract needy people who are slow to assume self-responsibility. On the other hand, care*giving* attracts psychologically strong people who are interested in becoming more whole; they are much more goal-oriented, and health-centered dentistry tends to align well with their lifestyle choices.

People who are stuck in too many caretaker roles (out of their need to create more efficiency in their life) attempt to fix other people's problems too quickly. Along the way, they inadvertently maintain the dependency state. In contrast, a caregiver will respectfully wait to be asked for help, as they respect interpersonal boundaries while simultaneously encouraging more self-responsibility.

With these concepts in mind, think about the patients of your practice, particularly those you'd rather avoid. The most likely reason you feel that way is that you have assumed a caretaker role in the relationship. Consequently, every time you engage them, you feel like you're required to surrender too much of yourself—for whatever reason, the relationship is highly transactional, and you have to barter off a little piece of yourself every time you get together. Here's the bottom line: How are you currently managing the number of caretaking relationships in your practice? Are there too many of them present for you to serve your other patients at the level they expect and deserve? If so, what strategies can you deploy to correct the imbalance between caretaking and caregiving in your practice?

135

If you look at the people around you and you don't get inspired, then you don't have a circle; you have a cage.

~Nipsey Hustle

Chapter 36
The Origin of Future Focusing

How intelligent must we be to succeed at relationship-based / health-centered dentistry? We often ask ourselves, "Am I smart enough to figure this out?" "Is there something wrong with me that's causing patients to reject my recommendations?" Frequent rejection causes us to build up a belief system based upon what we're experiencing instead of what's possible. In other words, we can quickly and subconsciously create a rut, similar to the one Harold Wirth described, and keep ourselves there via a limiting mindset.

On this topic, Bob Barkley said many dentists have a "slum mentality," referring to the work of Ben Singer, a Harvard PhD. Sociologist who rose to the top of academia out of the slums of South Boston. Most of Singer's childhood friends died from gang violence or were incarcerated, yet he went on to receive a PhD. and full professorship from one of the top universities in the world. Why? Answering that question was a driving force in Singer's life.

Bob Barkley read about Singer's work and applied it to dentistry. What did Singer learn? He learned that the most successful kids were those who were able to see themselves living differently in a future timeframe. Singer labeled the ability "future focus." Those who were able to future focus and envision a better life tended to make decisions that supported the attainment of their preferred future. In other words, they had constructive habits which motivated them to make better choices due to a vital goal kept top-of-mind. Over time, the habits, repeated over and over again, influenced their future more than almost anything else.

Conversely, Singer noticed that kids who were unable to imagine a better future for themselves tended to remain paralyzed in immaturity and self-destruction; they remained focused only on the day at hand and squandered their time, resources, energy, and money on feel-good, reactive pursuits. In other words, they weren't motivated to make sacrifices, plan, and delay gratification because it appeared pointless. Bob Barkley said dentists act in similar ways. Dentists who are able to imagine a values-driven, optimal future, commit to its attainment until it's achieved, and those who can't—don't.

Although we tend to equate intelligence with success, many studies demonstrate that beyond a certain level of competency, IQ has less and less influence over outcomes. Ben Singer proved it. The difference between succeeding at relationship-based/health-centered dentistry and failing lies in our ability to envision a future of choice and to become so motivated that we refuse to allow progress toward its attainment to be delayed. In other words, those who believe they can do it are the ones who are most likely to do it. It sounds pretty simple, but the process requires a lot of courage, sacrifice, commitment, and time.

If I distrust the human being, then I must cram him with information of my own choosing, lest he go his own mistaken way.

~Carl Rogers, PhD

Freedom to Learn, C.E.Merrill Publishing Co., 1969

Chapter 37
Charles Varipapa, D.D.S.

Those of you who know Charley Varipapa, D.D.S., know about his larger-than-life personality, combined with his ability to laugh at life, himself, and get you to laugh at yourself. And all the while, he sneaks in a funny story that's completely self-revealing while creating a learning moment that's all tied up in a belly laugh. I met Charley at The Pankey Institute in the late 90's. His stories and mindset had the whole class laughing and functioning in a cohesive fashion within just a few hours.

But there was a lot more going on than Charley joking around. When I pulled him aside during a wine-facilitated evening session, I learned more. It turned out Charley was dead serious about changing his very successful practice. He said that he was tired of "Happydale" and ready to move on.

"Happydale? I asked, "What's Happydale?" Charley said Happydale was when Mrs. Fellocotti (one of the many metaphorical people he invented to drive home a point) brings you a homemade cake because you've been so "nice" to her. "Yes," I said, "But what's wrong with that? And how is that related to Happydale?" "Well," Charley said, "Just because you're being nice and making a lot of money, doesn't mean your patients are becoming healthier and making good decisions. Mrs. Fellocotti still has that crappy partial denture, and she was happy because I agreed to repair her failing crown with an amalgam patch for the third time."

"Oh", I said, "I think I am beginning to understand—being nice has nothing to do with effective leadership." "Yep", Charley said, "Sometimes people have to learn about something they don't want to hear, because it's in their best interest, and Happydale is the place where that doesn't happen very often. That's why I'm here, to try and learn how to help my patients make better decisions."

We went on from our first meeting at to form the Bob Barkley Study Club a year later with M. Johnson Hagood, DDS. During that time, Charley sold his profitable practice in Southern Maryland and opened a new one in Old Town Alexandria, VA, based upon his new, more comprehensive, health-centered vision. The new practice was located in an attractive mid-1800's federal style row house in the center of the revitalized downtown. This time around, Charley only built two treatment rooms, one for himself and one for a part-time hygienist.

When you walked through the front door, you were immediately struck by its impeccable design; it felt like you had just entered Charley's home. Consequently, people went there to learn more about themselves through Charley's stories, analogies, and his strategically planned CoDiscovery experiences. In almost every case, they'd ask Charley to help them in the very best way possible. And as a result, his patients were much happier and healthier as the process allowed them to feel better about themselves and to function more optimally.

Chapter 38
Are you a Servant-Leader?

When we're the leader, the application of our wisdom is limited unless we've created a system based upon a developmental philosophy that brings out the best in others. Extensive knowledge, debt, and positional power cause many dentists to become overly focused on production and subsequently treat team members as a means to an end via carrots and sticks. That leadership style ramps up fear – fear of not hitting externally created goals, fear of losing out on bonuses, fear of failing, and as a consequence, team members stop feeling positive emotions, while their drive to improve, experiment, and learn fades.

That type of top-down leadership model, born out of the industrial age, is outdated and counterproductive if our goal is "high touch, high-tech," meaning a person-centered practice that brings all of today's advancements to the table. When we are overly focused on control and immediate goals, instead of on the development of our team members, we can easily shoot ourselves in the foot.

The key to success in the person-centered business model is to make certain we help each person on the Care Team feel purposeful, motivated, and energized because their daily work, albeit stressful at times, aligns with who they are inside. In other words, a developmental management style allows each person to bring their best self to the office each day. The best way to achieve a development-oriented management style is to assume the mindset of a servant leader. Servant leaders view their leadership role as being a facilitator, not as a controller. They want to experience team members thinking for themselves, taking calculated risks, exploring opportunities, and learning new skills. They know that when they create "win-win" employment arrangements, everyone benefits.

Servant-leaders operate from a place of humility as they know there is a tremendous amount of power in leveraging the expertise of team members who have "boots on the ground," as they are the ones with a unique perspective of problems faced on a daily basis. Consequently, servant leaders actively seek ideas and the potential contributions each person can bring to the table.

Servant leadership isn't submissive, rather it emerges out of clarified values and a vision. The servant leader has a crystal clear understanding of their *why,* and their responsibility to increase ownership, autonomy, and commitment among their followers (including patients). Servant leadership represents a deliberate movement away from what author Douglas McGregor called *Theory X*, an authoritative management style that holds a pessimistic view toward others. *Theory X* managers believe that employees aren't very motivated to do a good job because the primary reason they work is money and benefits. *Theory X*, therefore, easily leads into Taylorism, which is just another word for micromanagement.[81]

How can we view our team members more optimistically? By carefully selecting people we admire, individuals we can "love"— a willingness to invest ourselves in their success. Once we've assembled a core group of people we admire, we can ask how to best support them. Next, we listen carefully and gather up all of the necessary training and resources they need to optimally perform. Finally, we get out of the way and "manage by walking around." When we notice someone shining, we say something like: "I can't believe how masterfully you handled that situation, Kim; I don't think I could have ever managed that difficult situation so well!"

The servant leader strategy sounds simple: find the right people, put them on the proverbial "bus," and instead of telling them how to do their jobs, ask them how we can help them do their jobs better. But it's not simple—finding the right people, getting them to commit to our purpose and then remaining emotionally sensitive to what's happening around them requires a lot of work. This change in our leadership style creates a virtuous cycle. When each person is credited for their ideas and sees them put into practice, they want to share more, which causes us to admire them all the more. The net outcome is the creation of a significantly improved office culture that leads to increased office productivity as the increased level of interpersonal trust fosters more creative risk-taking and development.

The servant leadership style, based upon *Theory Y*, states when conditions are favorable, each (carefully selected) person finds work more appealing and they become more willing to use their natural ability to problem-solve and collaborate on commonly shared goals. When motivated through the *self*-rewards the servant-leader generates, Care Team members evolve into becoming better managers of themselves.

The servant leadership model is the engine at the center of every health-centered practice, wherein the hygienist becomes a self-leader, as does the administrative leader, the lead clinical assistant, the lab assistant, and so forth. By developing the strengths of all team members, we join forces and create outcomes many times greater than individual contributions could ever create on their own.

There is only one way to avoid criticism: do nothing, say nothing, and be nothing.

~Aristotle

Chapter 39
Happiness is a Choice

Given that the average dentist spends around 80,000 hours of their life working in their practice, it makes sense that they should try and discover ways to feel better about how we spend that time. But there's a paradox associated with this challenge. If we simply set a goal to feel happy most of the time, we'll fail miserably. That's because happiness is a fleeting state, and the more we chase it, the more elusive it becomes.

Happiness is not an emotion; emotions are instinctive and involuntary. Happiness is a *feeling*, and feelings always involve some level of cognitive evaluation. "It's a valuing function," said Carl Jung. Hence, happiness is the outcome of running an experience through our value system and deciding we enjoy it. So, a more appropriate goal is to make sure we are routinely engaged in personally meaningful work, and as an outcome, more joyful moments appear.

Emily Esfahani Smith, the author of *The Power of Meaning: Finding Fulfillment in a World Obsessed with Happiness,*[82] tells us that when we focus our time and energy on meaningful pursuits we are much more likely to feel an enduring sense of well-being. Why? Because we're focusing our time and energy on refining our experience instead of looking for ways to minimize the negative feelings generated by meaningless work. That's not to say that dentistry has to be the central purpose of our life, but it does support the idea that if we make our work in dentistry more congruent with who we are inside, we're more likely to improve, experience the positive feelings associated with mastery, and become more successful—we will create a positive reinforcement loop.

As a coach over the years to many dentists who expressed frustrations related to the latest trends: reduced insurance reimbursement, significantly higher overhead, staffing shortages, increased levels of rudeness and disregard from patients, higher levels of competition from corporate entities, and so forth, I often hear a desire to find greater meaning in work; I'm often told that the daily grind is taking too much of a toll on their soul.

Meaning Versus Happiness

Shawn Achor, author of the bestselling book *The Happiness Advantage*,[83] surveyed frustrated workers and found that 9 out of 10 stated they would swap a percentage of their lifetime earnings for the opportunity to be involved in more meaningful work. But what does that mean, and how is it related to happiness?

According to Roy Baumeister, PhD, three factors differentiate meaning from happiness:

1. Happiness correlates with our desire to feel satisfied, whereas meaning does not. "The frequency of good and bad feelings turns out to be irrelevant to meaning, which can flourish even in very forbidding conditions." (See Viktor Frankl)

2. Baumeister found that happiness relates directly to the here and now, while meaning "seems to come from assembling past, present, and future into some kind of coherent story." Our life can't feel meaningful unless our life trajectory makes sense to us. Hence, if we don't know who we are or where we're headed in life, we'll often end up in a state of anomie, a feeling of "alienation and purposelessness experienced by a person as a result of a lack of standards, values, or ideals." Baumeister's research[84] found that when we help others, it leads us toward feelings of meaningfulness, and when others help us to help others, it leads to even more happiness because the activity aligns so well with our value system. Relating all of this to dentistry: we all have physically and psychologically challenging days, but if we are able to move through those days with a group of people who share our values, pull in the same

direction, and make each day easier and more enjoyable, we become happy warriors.

3. Personal meaning is experienced when we behave in a fashion that's congruent with who we are inside. Unfortunately, that doesn't mean that we're going to be happy all of the time. Life isn't fair, and the sooner we accept that simple truth, the sooner we'll move closer to happiness and fulfillment, due to our refusal to assume a victim posture.

How to Begin

If you don't have a vision in mind of your preferred future in dentistry, you'll forever be searching for the proverbial needle in a haystack. Becoming clearer about who you are and what you want is key. And the more authentic you become, the more people align with your purpose and they evolve into *disciples* –people who share your passion for what you're doing. That magnifies your influence, and that's how we can make a living at health-centered dentistry –by trading meaningful services for money. From there, happiness is only just a short step away.

Chapter 40
Robert Insko, PhD

My personal story would be incomplete if I failed to mention an important relationship that helped catalyze my vision and encouraged me to proceed. In 1987, when I was struggling to find my footing in dentistry and simultaneously thinking of leaving the profession, I met Bob Insko. Bob was a retired Episcopal Priest who worked part-time as an associate rector in a small parish in Lexington, Kentucky. Bob had a PhD in Theology, a PhD in Psychology, and a PhD in Engineering. He was in his mid-70's, and ran a small counseling practice within walking distance of my home.

I had recently finished M. Scott Peck's *Road Less Traveled*, and the book's content had a tremendous impact on my life. In it, Peck suggested using counseling for the purpose of personal growth and development. I soon discovered a new way of thinking about the world, spirituality, myself, and my life through a helping relationship that led me into deep, meaningful conversations.

If I was in the mood to talk about dentistry as a career, Bob could do that. If I wanted to talk about God and scripture, Bob could do that. If I wanted to talk about my aspirations, failures, or psychological wounds, Bob could do that. He was my shaman for a couple of years, but his influence on my life is still with me today.

Through my relationship with Bob, I realized that I was important, capable, and courageous in spite of my doubts, flaws, and struggles. He encouraged me to keep asking the tough questions and to keep seeking answers. In other words, Bob encouraged me to keep growing, and how could I refuse such a challenge after being told that he'd started attending a Jewish Synagogue to better understand his Christian faith?

My reason for sharing this story with you is to encourage you to consider counseling, *but* when you do, make certain that you do it in a discriminating fashion. Don't enter a counseling relationship with the intention of "fixing" anything. Consider the possibility that counseling might be an excellent pathway through which you can discover better ways to develop yourself. There are many amazing counselors who have spent a significant part of their life asking the question *why,* and relentlessly pursuing the answer. At the same time, there are many counselors stuck in dogmatic approaches that will lead you toward more frustration and disappointment.

As dentists, we want our patients to be selective and discriminating, we want them to choose our practice for all the right reasons. Similarly, we need to be discriminating when it comes to the selection of our personal growth counselors.

As an added bonus, the non-judgmental relationship formed with Bob Insko taught me how to create similar relationships with my patients. Over time, I learned that the more I listened and the more I allowed my patients to listen to themselves, the more they changed for the better. Additionally, I discovered that I had to do very little convincing when I focused my attention on what the person was perceiving, what they were feeling, and what they *really* wanted. Finally, my most prominent memory associated with Bob isn't related to him telling me to do or think anything in particular; rather, it's a memory of Bob smiling and thus implying, "I am so pleased to see that you're finally starting to figure this out."

Chapter 41
The People Factor

L.D.Pankey commonly professed:

"I never saw a tooth walk into my office," which in its simplicity, is quite profound. Teeth are a lot of things – functional, sensory, and esthetic, but they can't drive, care for themselves, pay for their repair, or make themselves look better—only people can do that. So, if we don't understand how a person thinks or how to help them make better decisions, and therefore behave in a more sophisticated fashion regarding their health, then we'll forever be frustrated and under-compensated "tooth mechanics."

Avrom King liked to say, "The best run small practice will always be better at taking care of people than the best run large practice,"[85] which might be an obvious conclusion to those of us who run smaller practices, but why is that true?—the people factor. The larger an organization is, personnel-wise, the more managerial structures have to be put in place to control behavior and outcomes, which means systems and pre-programmed responses frequently replace intuition and finely-tuned decisions unique to each circumstance. In other words, the larger the organization, the more depersonalized it can become, although well-trained and sophisticated companies are very good at cloaking that truth via strategies, tactics, and technology.

For example, it's now quite common for corporate practices to have off-site practice administrators handle scheduling and other functions—people who don't live in the community, and who aren't emotionally invested in the future of the practice or its patients.

What's best for your future? That depends on what you want your future to look like. If your goal is to treat a maximal volume of insurance-influenced / associated patients, then you have no other choice but to build a large organization that's high in delegation and install a lot of command-and-control features. If your goal is optimal customer service and optimal outcomes focused on helping others make better decisions, then a smaller, more nimble, intuitive organization is needed.

Care team members are where the rubber meets the proverbial road, hence, they are a large part of how our "brand image" develops over time. If we put "C-players" on the front line, then the outcome is patients responding to C-player behavior. If we put real, authentic, values-clarified, highly skilled, and mission-centric people on the front line, then we get magic—meaning a much higher level of productivity per hour, a much higher level of patient satisfaction, greater profitability, and lower stress.

We can chase after the small stuff, or we can create bigger, more meaningful outcomes with fewer people and more intention. If we think we can chase after the small stuff as well as a finely tuned corporation that's industrialized the delivery of dental treatment down to every physical move, bulk material purchase, reimbursement rate negotiation, mass marketing discount, and the centralization of administration, then we're wrong. Admittedly, that's a hard lesson to learn when we're so busy that we barely have time to think about what's really happening in our practice.

Chapter 42
What Does Emotional Intelligence Look Like?

When we talk about Emotional Intelligence (EQ),[86] we're talking about emotional maturity and all of the benefits it brings into our life. EQ, unlike IQ, is developable but not easily or quickly. It's not found in the pages of a book, and it's not something we can memorize or come to understand after a great realization. Instead, it's a form of self-discipline that's most easily obtained through the modeling of emotionally mature parents or parental figures.

But what if our parents weren't emotionally mature, and as a result, we picked up some of their bad emotional habits? The good news is we can become more emotionally mature through self-reflection and a willingness to grow, learn, stumble, reframe, see things from other points of view, as well as through difficult experiences. It's a process that never ends, but as our emotional maturity grows, our ability to become more strategic, practical, and discerning accelerates. Emotional maturity can be observed in ourselves and others through habitual behavior patterns. The behavior patterns below are helpful for further self-development, but are also useful when hiring, when we need to understand a relationship on a deeper level, when we need to modify our leadership style, while parenting, and under many other circumstances.

The 12 Behaviors of an Emotionally Healthy Person

1. You don't blame-shift; instead, you own the problems and mistakes you helped create, or failed to address, in a timely fashion. Hence, you don't make others suffer the burden of your bad judgment or laziness. Instead, you face up to things, work on problem resolution, and move on.

2. You're willing to let yourself be selectively vulnerable. Life experiences have taught you that people can be deceptive, hurtful, hold hidden agendas—or worse, yet you understand the behavior of some people does not represent the behavior of all. Consequently, you become more discerning instead of cynical. The outcome is fewer but deeper friendships and associations based upon shared values and priorities. In other words, you know how to modulate and maintain interpersonal boundaries.

3. You're willing to be around people who hold different opinions, as long as they're able to do the same. Listening to and trying to understand other perspectives is how you learn, grow, change, or reinforce your beliefs regarding how the world works. Consequently, you read broadly, listen carefully, and dedicate yourself to discovering the truth.

4. Your life is expansive rather than limited and fixated upon maintaining the status quo. You know that the moment you stop learning, you'll stop growing, and when you stop growing, you start dying on the psychological level.

5. You don't expect others to anticipate your needs and desires. Instead, you state them clearly and make your agendas transparent so that others can choose to join you, help you, or move on.

6. You maintain low expectations, not because you think people will disappoint you, but because you understand how high expectations can sometimes be destructive in the long term. Hence, you're willing to be patient and wait people out – but only to the degree that being patient doesn't violate your boundaries.

7. You don't let past disappointments or injuries overly influence your future behavior. You may not have forgiven everyone for what they have done to you, but you can see the

experience as a harsh life lesson and then move on, having gained some wisdom from the process.

8. You are willing to forgive yourself for being imperfect. In other words, you don't hold grudges against yourself for bad decisions and undesirable outcomes. The key to success is learning, growing, strategically adjusting, and self-forgiveness.

9. Your goal isn't to be happy all the time; rather, it's to be content with what you have, what you've become, and where you're headed. There's much in life that you can't control, and believing there will be a time in your life when you'll never be sad, angry, frustrated, or disappointed is entirely unrealistic.

10. People don't easily trigger you. You understand you are driving the proverbial "bus," hence, there is a little voice in your head that says, "I need to slow down here... proceed with caution...don't overreact...I need to find a way to change the emotional tone of this situation." Since you're in touch with your emotions, you know there is always more to a story than what you currently know, and most of the time, when others are agitated, they aren't attacking you, they're reacting to a narrative in their head that may have very little to do with you.

11. You have learned that suppressing emotions is sometimes counterproductive. First, you let yourself feel it, then you decide on the appropriateness of expressing it at that moment. You know that if you allow the emotional valence of a situation to decrease before responding, you're a more effective leader. You also know emotions are like circus animals: they must be understood, respected, listened to, and strategically managed.

155

Opportunity is missed by most people because it is dressed in overalls and looks like work.

~Thomas Edison

Chapter 43
Brian Vence, D.D.S.

Brian Vence is a 1985 graduate of the University of Illinois, and practices in Oakbrook Terrace, Illinois[87]. Following graduation, Brian completed a GPR at the VA Wadsworth-UCLA hospital in addition to a mini-residency in TMD. Once his training was completed, Brian worked as an associate in several Southern California practices.

During that time, Brian became acquainted with Carl Rieder, one of the founders of the *American Academy of Esthetic Dentistry* and the *Newport Harbor Academy*. The *Newport Harbor Academy* met nine times a year and exposed Brian to the best dentistry in the world. Simultaneously, Brian became aware of the work of Avrom King, via newsletters and audio tapes. One of the tape series was titled, *Listening for Excellence,* wherein Avrom discussed how to interview patients for the purpose of more predictably identifying discriminating personality profiles, and their overall approach to life—"their philosophy," as Bob Barkley used to say.

Those experiences set Brian on a mission to find out how he could create outcomes similar to the top-level casework he was seeing at Academy meetings. The journey led Brian into learning how to stack porcelain and manage a significant part of the lab work himself, similar to Bob Winter (also an Academy member). Brian's father was a dental lab technician and owner, so he spent his formative years in the lab, starting out at the plaster bench.

Brian moved to the Chicago suburb of West Dundee in 1990, with a growing level of experience and a clear vision of where he wanted to take his practice. However, Brian was still uncertain about how to more predictably get his patients to proceed with comprehensive casework on a regular basis. Brian asked Aalt Brouwer, an associate of Avrom King, how to overcome that challenge. Aalt responded with a question, not an answer: "What kind of relationships do you have with your patients on the feeling level?" Alt's question puzzled Brian, who had up to that point thought feelings didn't belong in a dental practice. Over several years, Brian worked with Avrom King on a one-to-one basis and attended several three-day workshops. Over time, he progressively learned how to fully integrate CoDiscovery and the co-development of treatment plans into his practice model. However, that was only possible following a significant amount of work that eliminated a lot of Brian's subconscious, self-limiting behaviors. In combination, the focused efforts—understanding the technical aspects of dentistry on a very deep level, along with the psycho-social and leadership aspects—allowed Brian to consistently generate a significant amount of income out of a low-volume 900-square-foot office.

Brian recalled, "I remember shutting my feelings down as a kid so that I wouldn't get overly excited or anxious, and as a result, I had a tendency to project my feelings and agendas without realizing it." Brian's work with Avrom King and a private counselor led him toward understanding his emotions and managing his feelings in a much more sophisticated fashion. Once there, Brian was able to more accurately understand his patient's feelings, as well as see things from their perspective. That was key, because it allowed him to reorganize his communication style with each person to be centered around what *they* wanted, particularly *after* they had the opportunity to learn more about their situation and how they felt about it.

Brian's friendship with Carl Rieder led him into a relationship with E. Pat Allan, who invited him to attend an American Academy of Restorative Dentistry meeting. Brian was eventually asked to join the AARD and the American Academy of Esthetic Dentistry, both highly selective organizations associated with only the best-of-the-best.

By 2015, Brian had outgrown the West Dundee facility and resolved the problem by purchasing a practice in Oakbrook

Terrace. He merged the two practices together, which allowed him to spread out in a more appropriately designed facility in the same building as his periodontist George Mandalaris. Brian works closely with Lynn Turk, R.D.H. who functions as his full-time *Patient Care Coordinator*. Together, they run a sophisticated ten-step new patient integration process. Brian said, "We have six steps before we sit down and develop a treatment plan, because it usually takes that long to get the person to the point—education and understanding-wise—that they're able to participate in an intelligent fashion."

Brian's systems and highly coordinated team allowed him to double production without significantly increasing the number of patients he sees each day. With Lynn completing initial interviews, Brian is free to focus his attention on discovering *the meaning of potential treatment to each person*. He believes that most people present with one of four primary meanings that motivate their behavior:

1. The desire for Symptomatic relief of a disease process or problem

2. Social meaning – how they feel about how they think others perceive them

3. Personal meaning – a personal goal, such as feeling more "whole," or looking better

4. Familial meaning – a family member is pushing them to take action

Brian assumes a different communication strategy for each situation, with some cases leading to the conclusion that it might be best if they decide to *not* work together, as his focus is primarily on the creation of stable, long-term health through comprehensive, health-centered strategies. Brian said:

I want my patients to develop a personal vision of how they want to appear and how they want to lower their risk of encountering

problems in the future. CoDiscovery is a big aspect of how we do that. We try to weave the meaning of the treatment into the task at hand. We co-discover how the person's current condition evolved, but we also discuss where they want to go. All of that occurs within a helping relationship that eventually leads into a discussion about what I can provide for them that will look great and last a long time. To me, CoDiscovery is like a boat—it's the vehicle. Let's say I have a boat that can take us across Lake Michigan. The first thing we need to figure out is: Where we are starting from?

Are we in Chicago? Are we in Milwaukee? Are we in Green Bay? Next, we need to figure out where we want to go: Do we want to go to South Holland? Do we want to go up to Traverse City? Next is: Why are we going? That's a critically important thing to figure out, because if we can't clearly define the "why," then it will be difficult for the person to get behind the "what" required to get them to their end-goal. Not to sound too corny, but I kind of see myself as both a Shaman and a Sherpa in each new relationship. In the Shaman role, I try to address the meaning side –I try to help each person discover why they want to do something. For instance, some people are very committed to doing things for their kids and their family, but they aren't very good at doing things for themselves. So, sometimes a spouse is the motivator in the background that's pushing the person to take action. And that can be a big hurdle to get around to successfully assist the person in the process of becoming more whole. The other part of the equation is the "what": What do we need to do to get the person where we want to go? So, the Shaman role is centered around better understanding the "why" (which can evolve in some cases over time as we get farther along in the treatment process), and the Sherpa role is related to discovering the "what": If this is where you are now, what is going to be required to get you where you need to go? Improved health, better appearance, improved self-esteem—whatever that particular person wants as the outcome of their treatment journey.

Currently, Brian is a leader in the use of SFOT (surgically facilitated rapid orthodontic therapy), which can be used to significantly improve dental arch form and as well as increase bone mass. He is a strong advocate for coordinated multi-disciplinary care, and is the co-editor of *Surgically Facilitated Orthodontic Therapy, An Interdisciplinary Approach* with George Mandalaris. Brian is also a frequent co-presenter at Bob Barkley Study Club CoDiscovery workshops, where he takes people through his CoDiscovery systems and processes.

Chapter 44
The Human Mind and Case Acceptance

Our brain is a predictive machine that's always turned on. To a large degree, it operates like the autocomplete function on a phone—it's constantly trying to guess the next word or intention. It will attempt predictions on several levels: threat, meaning, in-tribe or out-tribe, and attractiveness. To do that, it compares sensory information with memories of similar situations and patterns. The more negative the memories, the more negative the prediction, and the more conservative or defensive the response. Additionally, it likes to stack the odds 4:1 in its favor, meaning that our brain tends to predict adverse outcomes four times more often than positive outcomes when it's in an unfamiliar situation.

These inherent mental functions influence most of our first impressions and decision-making, so it's useful to understand how they influence patient behavior. Unless we enter a new relationship with a stellar reputation, the odds are 4:1 against our ability to advance a health-centered agenda, particularly when a person has a negative history associated with dentistry. That's a steep hill, yet we tend to ignore it. The best way to overcome the odds is to strategically allow trust to develop through the creation of simple, low-risk proposals that lead to strong positive feelings and future memories – that's what Bob Barkley, Harold Wirth, L.D. Pankey, Bill Strupp, Gary DeWood, Mary Osborne, Mike Schuster, Charlie Varipapa, Rich Green, Lynn Carlisle, Brian Vence, Fred Lima, and many others did—or are currently doing.

For example, would you agree to hire a contractor to build your dream home without first spending a significant amount of time researching the quality of their previous work, listening to how others felt about their process, and personally sizing them up? Would you hire a financial planner to manage all of your assets without first doing a similar amount of research? Probably not, but for some reason, we dentists want to believe that when a person is in need of extensive oral rehabilitation or restoration, they'll be ready to make a multi-thousand-dollar decision within an hour or so of meeting us simply because we have a DDS or DMD hanging off the end of our name.

Generally speaking, people don't respond well to that kind of approach—recall the Avrom King (I fear for your soul) story. According to Mike Schuster, comprehensive case acceptance rates hover around 35% for the average practice, because it involves the onboarding of too much information too quickly, from a virtual stranger who has yet to prove their trustworthiness. Bob Barkley's CoDiscovery/CoDiagnosis/Success Planning process helps to significantly increase case acceptance rates because it aligns well with how the mind works:

1. Trust (enhanced by how we structure our new patient experience)

2. Learn (facilitated by *how* we teach and share information)

3. Decide (facilitated by how well we align what we are teaching to what they want)

4. Commit (driven by the person's beliefs and values)

5. Follow through (sustained by our support and reconfirming what they want)

Chapter 45
The Sympathetic Nervous System Isn't Very Sympathetic

Our sympathetic nervous system – our subconscious, primal "fight or flight" self-preservation system,[88] doesn't give a damn about what we think – or what anyone else thinks, for that matter. And that's because this critically important system, mediated by our midbrain, evolved (from an evolutionary biology standpoint) at least two hundred million years before the cerebral cortex came on the scene. In other words, feelings and memory-based perceptions drove behavior long before significant cognition emerged. Consequently, a significant part of our brain didn't evolve for the purpose of higher math, understanding physics, or philosophizing about the meaning of life—it's primarily there to keep us alive for another day.

If we want to refine our thinking, modify our beliefs, and make better and more sophisticated health-centered decisions, our "lower" instinctive desires must be addressed. In other words, if our "lower" brain thinks there's an existential threat (real or imagined), it isn't going to be concerned with how others feel, nor will it be interested in our long-term needs. That's why all health-centered relationships—relationships that have as their core purpose the advancement of health in others—require a special kind of interpersonal experience, an experience that needs to be repeated over and over again until safety is *felt*. In other words, when we repeatedly create a safe-feeling environment, it supports better long-term decision-making because it satiates the self-preservation instinct—it ramps down the sympathetic nervous system activity, which then allows the parasympathetic system to predominate (relax, rest, learn, and make more values-based decisions).

Similarly, when a doctor and team are stressed and distracted, they aren't very attuned to how their patients are feeling, what they're perceiving, and what they may or may not be learning. A patient's limbic system has good reason to perceive that type of behavior as a potential threat, so it will default to a self-preservation mode that skips right past good decision-making.

We suffer not from events in our lives, but from our judgment about them.

~ Epictetus

Chapter 46
Shame Drives Behavior

Shame is the most powerful of our negative emotions, because it's a social emotion. Shame is a psychological force that can shape daily behavior or the arc of an entire life. It's so powerful that most people avoid shame at any cost, and consequently fail to learn that the root might be based on a distorted perspective of reality.[89]

Most patients approach dentists with an expectation of being judged, combined with feelings of inadequacy. That can easily trigger shame, which shuts down their ability to learn and make values-based decisions. Shame is driven by memories linked to powerful emotions associated with rejection. The memories, held in the hippocampus and neocortex, are immediately available for recall when a new experience resembles a threatening pattern from the past. The old memory triggers a refractory period that can lead to self-contempt (the important distinction between guilt and shame is the following: Guilt = *I feel bad* because I made a mistake, but I'm ok. Shame = *I am bad* because I made a mistake = *I am a mistake*). In other words, new experiences trigger old feelings linked to old memories that are projected onto the current circumstance. The outcome can create a sense of helplessness and hopelessness. Chronic feelings of that nature cause a person to believe the same negative things will keep happening over and over again. When a patient has a lot of negative memories and is confronted by an insensitive dental team, they can easily think: "Why don't I just have all of my teeth taken out? Even though I'd rather not, it will eliminate all future problems and all of these stressful and embarrassing moments. They said they have sedation, maybe it won't be too bad!"

That's how the brain works. *It's designed to make immediate issues more important than long-term health unless the process is overridden* by conscious thinking. That's why Bob Barkley said,

"We have to get people to think differently." Our brain can hurt us when it's attempting to protect us, as it has no long-term perspective when threatened—even if the threat occurred twenty years ago.

Helping others make complex, long-range decisions requires us to move patients past their current level of awareness and preoccupations toward a vision of something significantly better. On the neuroscience level, that means we need to help each person move away from the negative emotions and memories that are holding them back from making better decisions. Bob Barkley designed CoDiscovery to do that—to move a person away from *deductive* thinking toward *inductive* thinking. <u>Inductive thinking is primarily a right hemisphere function and is self-narrative driven.</u> Bob called that self-narrative "future focusing," a term that he learned from Ben Singer, PhD.

Chapter 47
Bob Barkley and the Learning Ladder

Bob Barkley felt it was important to determine where a person was on the *Learning Ladder*[90] as it helped facilitate each per-son's progress toward making better decisions, and therefore taking appropriate action. Bob knew motivation was an "inside job," something that he could only promote—but not give to another person. Bob observed that his patients were frequently stuck at the *belief level*—they understood they had a problem, yet weren't committed to taking the necessary action to resolve it. Bob said, "If you want to motivate someone, the most you can do is stimulate them to think more for themselves in a future-focused fashion, and that will hopefully begin the process of the person motivating themselves." Bob believed it was the dentist and care team's responsibility to catalyze the formation of a commitment to take action. He said, "A subtle alchemy is required to take a belief and turn it into a commitment. The essential distinction is that a commitment becomes a viable part of an individual's lifestyle, whereas a belief is not yet as integral to the individual."

So, you can see that Bob functioned in a very strategic fashion with his patients—hence, there was never anything random about how he communicated. He made sure he knew where each person was on the learning ladder, and then focused his attention on trying to find out *why* the person wasn't committing to the pursuit of stable, long-term health. Once Bob understood *why* a person was "stuck," he'd work on ways to help them around the barriers: Was there something they didn't understand? Did they believe that the decision to proceed wasn't in their long-term best interest? Were they not ready on a financial level? Did they lack a long-term vision for a preferred health and future? Bob also understood that the process and the ability to follow through might take 2-3 years for some people.

Steps on the Learning Ladder:

7. Sustained goal-oriented behavior

6. Willingness to pay the prices: time, energy, and money

5. Belief that the problem can be successfully resolved

4. Mindset shift: "I think I need to do something about this problem."

3. Realization that the problem is relevant

2. Awareness

1. Unawareness

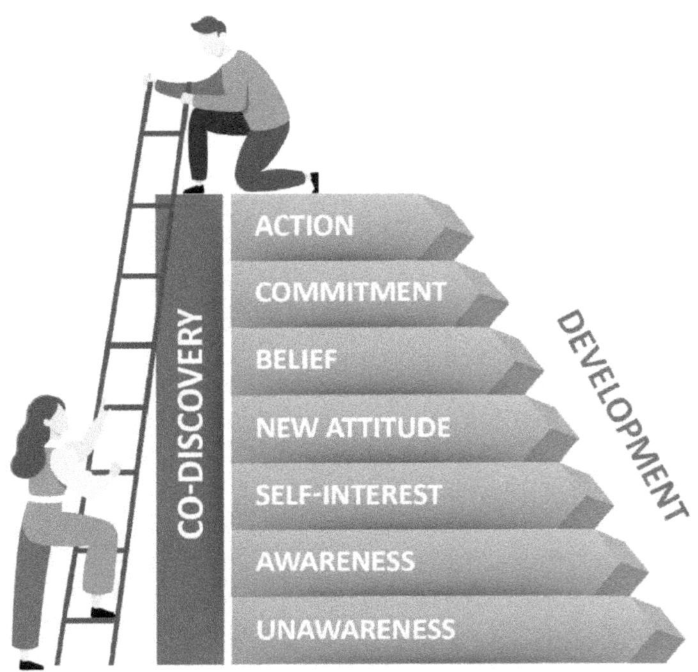

Chapter 48
Johnson Hagood, D.D.S.

M. Johnson Hagood is a 1986 graduate of East Carolina University.[91] He attended ECU with the intention of applying to medical school. His GPA and MCAT scores weren't strong enough to make the cut, so he shared his dilemma with his academic advisor, who suggested he consider dental school because of his artistic talents. Johnson then applied to the University of North Carolina School of Dentistry. The process required a gap year, so he moved to Chapel Hill to build his resume and make some money.

He landed a job in the dental school's TMJ pain clinic, in addition to waiting tables at McCarthy's restaurant. While there, Steve Hart,[92] came in for lunch. The serendipitous meeting would end up changing the course of Johnson's life. That conversation led Steve to make a job offer after discovering Johnson had recently applied to dental school.

Once in dental school, Johnson said that he sailed through *"without taking it too seriously."* Even with his limited knowledge, Johnson could see that Steve's practice was quite sophisticated. He soon learned that a lot of Steve's advanced training had come from *The Pankey Institute,* where he was an instructor. "I knew I wanted to go to *The Pankey Institute* before I graduated," he said.

After dental school, Johnson set up a scratch one-chair practice in Virginia Beach. "I thought I could pull off trying to be a combination of Steve Hart and Frank Spear," he said. That turned into a fateful decision, since Johnson did not participate in dental insurance. Regardless, Johnson put his shoulder to the task and attended *The Pankey Institute*, joined the AACD, and substantially elevated his clinical skills.

At that time, the author met Johnson at a photography course he was teaching. After that day, we made plans to start a behaviorally-oriented study club that would later be named *The Bob Barkley Study Club*. Bob Barkley Study club events and many conversations helped Johnson to successfully integrate CoDiscovery, CoDiagnosis, and co-treatment planning into his practice.

However, in spite of his exceptional skill set and growing behavioral skills, Johnson struggled to find enough discriminating patients willing to leave their insurance network. Linda Miles told him, "You know Johnson, your main problem is that you're trying to sell filet mignon in a hamburger town." In spite of the challenges, Johnson completed a number of beautiful aesthetic cases (sometimes at no fee) and became an accredited member of the *American Academy of Cosmetic Dentistry*. He then passed the Florida Board exam on his first try and moved to Vero Beach in 2001. The practice Johnson purchased was insurance-centric, in combination with low fees for everyone else. The dentist was older, and the average client had very little interest in fine esthetic dentistry, much less paying a proper fee to receive it. Regardless, Johnson put his shoulder to the task, made the math work, and slowly transitioned the practice toward comprehensive and esthetic dentistry. "In the beginning, I had a lot of patients who wouldn't even buy green bananas," Johnson said.

Over time, Johnson earned the respect of the best specialists in the region. Additionally, his reputation for top-level esthetic outcomes through collaboration with Rick Shafer, C.D.T., at Bayview Lab expanded.

Currently, Johnson has a thriving practice that receives referrals from Pankey and AACD-affiliated doctors around the country. Additionally, he is a fellow of the AACD, a visiting faculty member of *The Pankey Institute,* and a Pankey Scholar. (Pankey Scholar status is the equivalent of passing a specialty board exam, in combination with a deep dive into how a person runs their practice and life on both the behavioral and financial levels.)

Johnson has also won several regional art shows. The walls of his office are covered with his artwork and function as nice conversational segues into how artistic abilities translate over to esthetic dentistry.

Dr. David Swan wrote:

In my role as the coordinator for the Pankey Scholar program, I've been fortunate to be in the room for nearly 300 Scholar presentations. Johnson Hagood has a rare combination of talent and humility, coupled with a solid work ethic, personal transparency, and an intentional balance of work, play, love, and worship, that embodies the definition of eudaemonia—human flourishing. It's important in our profession to have role models who have stayed true to their vision and made a success of it. In today's world, it's even more important to know that there might be another way, a better way. Johnson has worked hard to incorporate the philosophical, behavioral, and technical competencies it takes to be a master dentist.

Chapter 49
Wants Versus Needs

A need is a feeling that you want to be rid of, and once rid of it, you don't want that feeling again. On the other hand, when a person values something they want more of it.[93]   ~Charles Sorenson, PhD

It's a simple truth that when confronted with a decision, and we're clear about what we value, we are less price-sensitive: "I feel like I should start taking better care of myself. I know this is going to be expensive, but I feel strongly that it's the right thing to do." Conversely, when we're confronted by a decision that involves something we don't value very highly, we become price sensitive: "Does my insurance cover that? Is it going on sale any time soon? Is there a cheaper alternative?"

Values belong to the world of feelings and beliefs, and therefore, they aren't entirely in the world of consciousness. Consequently, the extent to which a new patient experience is directed toward uncovering and exploring values, the more we can help them move beyond fee and toward a more sophisticated decision-making process. Values and feelings are associated with the *qualitative* aspects of life. Cost, on the other hand, is *quantitative*. So, exploring values and priorities is often an open, creative, and possibilities-oriented process, whereas a focus on cost involves a much more objective conversation.

When cost is analyzed too early in a new relationship, particularly when a person has a lot to learn about their situation, it tends to shut down creative problem-solving (*Note*: This is *why* Brian Vence has six steps before he starts to treatment plan a complex case with a patient). Hence, when values, priorities, and goals *aren't* clarified on the front end of a problem-solving discussion (before costs and "coverage" are discussed), then the human mind naturally defaults to *a fear of loss*. In heuristics, fear of loss is called "scarcity bias." The key to improving case acceptance for health-centered dentistry is to avoid triggering scarcity bias, and that's accomplished by structuring the new patient process in such a way that each person is allowed an appropriate amount of time to consider qualities (values/feelings/goals/preferred future), *before* the conversation moves into an analysis of quantities (time/energy/money) required to complete the treatment in the most appropriate fashion.

That is not to say every time things are done in this order, cost is eliminated as a variable—that's unrealistic. Instead, the goal is to avoid setting up a scenario wherein a person's thinking automatically defaults to a cost analysis: "Is that covered?" *before* they have thoroughly considered the *value* of the treatment relative to their long-term health and well-being goals: "What's in my best interest health-wise? How can I make this best choice work out financially?"

That's the purpose of CoDiscovery, and why Bob Barkley told his patients, "Let's make quality the constant, and time the variable," meaning: let's first figure out the right thing to do, *and then* determine the best time to do it (which might mean that the patient will need to delay definitive treatment until they can afford it), instead of compromising their health outcome by encouraging them to accept a lower quality, less-expensive option. In those cases, a stabilization plan is created that allows the patient to be "held" until they're ready to proceed. In other words, the optimal goal (vision) isn't compromised, the *timing* of the execution is delayed.

Imagine a world where orthopedic surgeons say to their patients, "I have three different quality levels of prosthetic knees. The best one works out very nicely, the next one works out some of the time, and the cheapest one breaks frequently. Which one would you like me to use? Your insurance company won't pay for the best type of prosthetic knee.

I cannot teach anybody anything, I can only make them think.

~Socrates

Chapter 50
The Psycho-Social Nature of Patient Decisions

We want to be liked and accepted, and we want to make good decisions, so when we're confronted with a problem or a challenge that we know very little about, we use a cognitive-social strategy by:

Asking friends for advice

Observing what other people do

Reading testimonials and comparing them to our experiences

And then we: Respond emotionally with the support of a few assumptions

Psychologists tell us that we base most of our decisions on incomplete fact-gathering processes that are tainted by various forms of cognitive bias. In fact, our decision-making process is sometimes completely devoid of facts. We see this phenomenon in dentistry when a patient enters a practice with preconceived notions developed from their social environment or through inaccurately recalled memories.

Some people function off of ***survivorship bias***, which is a natural tendency to assume that the most visible people/businesses in the marketplace are the most skilled and successful (see Aspen Dental® and other mass-marketed companies). In other words, in the popularity contest of life, less visible options aren't even considered by most people. A marketing executive once told me, "If you aren't in the top three, relative to top-of-mind, you might as well not exist."

Our patients can also be motivated by ***loss aversion***, which refers to the brain's preference to avoid losses when making acquisitions. In other words, we have a natural tendency to seek out bargains instead of focusing our attention on quality, *unless* we have entered into the decision-making process *primed* to seek out the quality choice: "I want a Rolex watch. I know they cost a lot more than watches, and they don't keep time any better, but I like the way they look, how other people admire them, and how they hold their value." "I want to eat dinner at Anthony's Restaurant. I know that it will cost twice as much to eat there as at every other restaurant in town, but I really enjoy going there. Anthony's service, food, and ambiance are second to none, and I'm never disappointed—I'm worth it."

An example of this phenomenon in dentistry: When patients pay with *happy dollars*, meaning situations where the patient values the outcome more than they value holding onto their money. In dentistry, overcoming the tendency toward loss aversion requires the establishment of a strong, positive *brand expectation* with lots of quality themes that appeal to a person's long-term priorities.

On the other hand, the perceived value of a discounted fee is primarily a *quantitative* mental phenomenon that leverages loss aversion. That's why dental insurance is used as a tool to lure people toward a practice. Is this a strategy that can be used to build a practice? Absolutely yes! — but the people attracted by the strategy will often be loss-aversion motivated *while still expecting a high-quality outcome*. When a practice is unable to deliver high-quality care at a low price, a significant number of its patients will become frustrated and start looking for a new office. In that way, discounting destabilizes a practice. Conversely, if a practice chooses to focus its attention on quality (they decide to use a value-added marketing strategy instead of a loss aversion strategy), then discounts are unnecessary. Just like a well-regarded restaurant, most patients will keep returning because their expectations are always met or exceeded. Thus, new arrivals to the practice enter for the right reasons—and stay! (See the Johnson Hagood practice development story as an excellent example).

Patients are also influenced by what is known as the **availability heuristic**, which is a mental trigger that causes them to assume the first thing that comes to mind is the most relevant. For instance, when people think of dental insurance company X, they are primarily thinking about saving money and aren't considering the fact that policy is limited and third-party restricted. Dental insurance companies are excellent at leveraging the availability heuristic despite the fact that they generate a tremendous amount of frustration and disappointment. How can these insurance companies be so successful?—by leveraging massive marketing budgets that continuously reinforce a quality narrative that frequently isn't true.

Finally, patients tend to use *confirmation bias* and search for information that confirms their preexisting beliefs while ignoring or devaluing information that contradicts them. An example of confirmation bias is when a patient believes all dentists will hurt them or that all out-of-network dentists are shady, unreasonable, and uncustomary! Insurance companies use confirmation bias to manipulate consumer behavior and discourage people from seeking out-of-network assistance.

You can now see that the psycho-social nature of our relationships before, during, and after treatment are complex and full of potential cognitive distortions when we fail to proactively manage them.

If I accept the other person as something fixed, already diagnosed and classified, already shaped by his past, then I am doing my part to confirm this limited hypothesis. If I accept him as being in a process of becoming, then I am doing what I can to confirm or make real potentialities.

~Carl R. Rogers, PhD

On Becoming a Person

Chapter 51
You Must Demonstrate Ethical Proof

Dental practices that fail to communicate their philosophy, inadvertently encourage patients to base their decisions on empirical evidence and emotion. In other words, patients can only make fully-informed decisions when they link what they've learned to their values and longer-term priorities. That's why the decision to restore the mouth to optimal health, function, and appearance is difficult for the average patient—the average person in the average practice can't conceptualize the long-term value of proper restoration relative to the near-term cost. A powerful preventive-restorative practice philosophy (meaning restoration to optimal health, form, and function and *not* just repairs that attempt to stabilize a declining status quo) is the compelling narrative that helps bring the *why* to the *how*. Without the *why*, the average person will focus their attention on loss aversion (how much time, energy, and money will I lose?). That's a form of deductive thinking that is not future-focused. Example: When we use an intra-oral camera to show a broken posterior tooth due to the progressive loss of anterior guidance, we are only showing the symptom – not the cause. If we fail to help the person learn about the destructive process that led to the symptom, we failed to put the issue into the right context; we didn't create the opportunity for the person to conceptualize that individual teeth are part of a complex, interrelated system. The outcome: the person only agrees to repair problems as they arise and/or do "what my insurance covers." On the other hand, if we take the time to show articulated models and then demonstrate that the fractured tooth is *a symptom of a dysfunctional system*, then the clinical findings take on a different meaning to the person, and their decision-making is significantly influenced by the new perspective.

Communicating our preventive-corrective practice philosophy, provides what Aristotle called *ethical proof*, a critical component of the triad of proofs—ethical, emotional, and logical—necessary to create a compelling argument. Complex, progressive dental problems require compelling arguments if we want the person to say "yes" to proper corrective treatment.

Lastly, a practice philosophy must be internalized by everyone on the care team. In other words, everyone must *be it* and not just *say it,* as discriminating patients—the individuals who are most likely to say *yes* to a comprehensive treatment plan—can sense incongruity between a message and the heart of the messenger. When they sense incongruity, they are much more likely to decline, seek another opinion, or delay. *Being it* is only possible through values-clarifying conversations and behavior that occurs continuously within the care team. *Being it*—the demonstration of ethical behavior—is therefore essential if we want to build a practice that's capable of routinely helping others properly address their complex problems. Once a truly helping relationship is established through the utilization of Aristotle's *proofs*, a confirming nod, a brief clarification, a smile, or a hug is often all that's needed to get the person to proceed forward with a mutually agreed-upon plan. Hence, there is no need to "sell" beyond authentically demonstrating who we are, what we believe in, and how we do things.

Chapter 52
Disequilibria

We are a living paradox: we're alive because we're constantly dying—the cells of our body come and go—yet we remain! A similar paradox exists on the psychological level. We can only grow and prosper psychologically if we're willing to let go of outdated beliefs and understandings—we must be willing to allow some of them to die off, and be replaced by more accurate, effective, and meaningful understandings.

Our new patients are often faced with a similar situation, part of their physical self is damaged, failing, or dying, and that's why they've come through our door. But what do they believe about what happened and why? When a person's beliefs are significantly out of sync with the reality of their problem, it creates a lot of stress and anxiety because they don't know who or what to believe.

The great developmental psychologist Jean Piaget, PhD.,[94] called these situations "disequilibria," a term that describes the psychological state of a person whose belief system and subsequent behavior pattern isn't able to consistently produce a desired outcome (Albert Einstein called the constant repetition of these patterns "insanity"). Under those circumstances, the person is forced to make a choice:

1. Continue what they are doing and hope for a different outcome

2. Change what they believe, organize a new strategy, and behave differently

Thus, during periods of disequilibria, a person will either learn and grow, or they will cling even harder to their beliefs through the denial of responsibility, assumption of a victim posture, or blame-shifting.

How we work with patients at these (potentially) paradigm-shifting moments has a tremendous influence on the future of our practice. For example, if we rescue a person too quickly from their problems (which is easy to do because of the way dental insurance is structured) we bypass their ability to reorganize their belief system and behavior. Hence, we undercut their progress toward making more health-centered decisions. Functionally, we allow them to repeat the *insanity* of the past because we're both easily and quickly financially rewarded. That's how codependency relationships operate, the low-hanging fruit of a person's simple and apparent needs are quickly harvested without any significant attempt to engage the person's thinking and behavior on a deeper level.

There are many situations in dentistry where learning on the part of the patient isn't crucial to the advancement of their long-term health: an old filling breaks, a person falls and chips a tooth, and so forth. Yet, most problems in dentistry—if we take the time to fully understand them—*do* require the patient's involvement if stable, long-term health is the goal. And that's where CoDiscovery fits into the picture. CoDiscovery allows each person to see their challenges in a more relevant way so they can attach more meaning to what they've learned. Significant meaning is what modifies beliefs, causes new commitments to be made, and facilitates better outcomes. On the other hand, when a person repeatedly fails to learn and grow, it can lead to neuroticism, dependency, frustration, and confrontations.

Questions:

1. How many times have we been the unwitting participant in the failure of a patient to make better decisions because we undermined their ability to learn and grow due to the way that we teach, or our need for short-term income?

2. How many times have we become too impatient and tried to resolve a person's problem for them, only to see it re-emerge again and again due to a lack of behavioral change?

Bob Barkley had a developmental mindset similar to what Stephen Covey referred to as "The Law of the Farm"—you reap what you sow. Bob felt that most people were unable to make good decisions early in a relationship (particularly when they faced complex problems), so he focused on how people learn and, therefore, *how to best facilitate more effective learning*. Bob believed that patients change their attitude toward their problem at their own pace, and that most make better decisions over time when the care team is comprised of effective teachers. Better teaching leads to more meaningful learning, and less disequilibria; less disequilibria leads to more goal-oriented thinking and better outcomes.

Chapter 53
The Insurance Issue

Insurance is meant to be financial protection against the occurrence of infrequent, catastrophic events. Originally, insurance was designed to compensate for large-scale losses associated with fire, flood, and theft. Later, the concept of was extended into Life, Auto, and Health. However, the function of "dental insurance" is quite different in that it represents *limited payments for frequent occurrences, with no provision for protection against catastrophic loss.* Hence, dental insurance is a misnomer for a tax-free benefit of employment.

Optimally, employers would like for their employees to have a dental benefit plan and never use it, because its use causes time away from work. Consequently, dental benefit plans tend to be chosen by employers based on cost, not on quality. Employers simply want to be able to tell prospective employees, "We offer dental insurance," *not* "We offer a dental health plan that will help you maintain your oral health over your lifetime."

Because most dental plans are minimal in coverage and restricted, it falls upon the care team to clarify the misconceptions. And if the misconceptions aren't proactively addressed, then the "subscriber" will function based on many wrong assumptions. When wrong assumptions are discovered after the fact, patients conclude that it's the dental office's fault that their coverage is so limited. In those cases, the dental office, for whatever reason, failed to get in front of the person's misconceptions (a thankless and often futile task). When a dental office has to clarify an insurance-created misunderstanding that's financially impacting a patient, it's often perceived as an excuse, incompetence, or worse.

Dealing with financial misconceptions after the fact must therefore be avoided at every turn, as patients need to know what to expect.

When misconceptions frequently occur, the confusion and disappointment damage or destroy trust in the entire practice.

Additionally, the "insurance" company's goal is to limit compensation, because the more it limits, the more profitable the plan. The same holds true for "non-profit" companies whose C-suite executives make millions of dollars a year and oversee the management of vast investment portfolios.

Because dental insurance company motives are primarily associated with *their* financial goals, they have every reason to support dentists who are willing to go along with their agendas, and they have every reason to undermine (directly and indirectly) dentists who refuse to cooperate. Clearly, that scenario puts "non-participating" dentists at a significant disadvantage, as dental insurance profitability goals are achieved primarily through communication with subscribers—sometimes before, and sometimes after treatment has been rendered. That's how they control their financial exposure—by intervening in the doctor/patient decision-making process; They want to weigh-in on most decisions and impose *their* standard of care (least expensive alternative treatment).

Chapter 54
UCR: Usual, Customary, Reasonable?

Dental insurance companies use the term "UCR" when communicating with subscribers. UCR is a percentage (commonly 80%) of the average of regional fees as reported by dentists. Many dentists don't annually update their fees or submit them to the insurance companies, so the computation is low to begin with, but the main take-away is that *no fee is UCR unless it's around 20% below the regional average.*

UCR is a *euphemism* for what an insurance company is willing to pay a dentist under contract. As stated, the amount paid represents a statistical calculation that has nothing to do with the quality of care, skill of the dentist, overhead of the office, quality of the care team, etc. As a result, contractually obligated dentists are forced to modify their business model to fit with the reimbursement model. That is accomplished primarily three ways:

1. Working faster, increasing "economy of scale," and increasing facility utilization

2. Increasing volume by "selling" dentistry through emotional manipulation

3. Reducing overhead by using less expensive materials, bulk purchasing, employment of lower-quality staff, outsourcing administrative functions, etc.

The above strategies worked well for many practices until insurance companies started to significantly *reduce* compensation. For example, an insurance company recently reduced compensation by 13% in California and 15% in Washington State while giving C-suite executives massive bonuses. Compensation reduction, combined with skyrocketing inflation and educational debt, fuels practice consolidation and industrialization. Consequently, there will be fewer solo practices and significantly more corporate ownership in the future. Thriving solo practices will be run by dentists who provide a philosophy of care and a quality of service that's *distinctly* better than what's offered elsewhere in the marketplace.

As perceived by the general public and *not just* by those who are running the practice.

The less a service is perceived to be a need, the more profitable it can be provided to those who want it.

~Avrom E. King

Chapter 55
What Message Do Your Fees Convey?

We rarely consider that our fees are a form of communication,[95] but when we allow a third party to set our fees, we are allowing them to communicate on our behalf. Is that a good thing? It depends on our goals: When a person buys a #3 Meal at McDonalds™, it has an associated price and an associated expectation. Who sets the expectations?—the McDonalds™ corporation. When a person purchases services from our practice, who sets the price, and who sets the expectations? Those are important questions to answer. Is our service quality set to match third-party compensation levels, or is our first consideration figuring out the best way to deliver optimal value *and then* setting a price that assures our ability to sustain the creation of that value day in and day out?

Dental insurance also tends to disrupt the natural order of social interactions, thereby complicating financial transactions in dentistry. Economist Thomas Sowell said, "Prices are important not because money is considered paramount but because prices are a fast and effective conveyor of information through a vast society in which fragmented knowledge must be coordinated." If we fail to take the lead in the minds of our current and prospective patients, then the lowest common denominator – price, rules the day due to the always-present scarcity bias built into our neurobiology. In other words, if we fail to create a solid and easily comprehended *superior value proposition*, we'll be perceived as being of no greater value than everyone else with a D.D.S. or D.M.D. after their name. In the world of marketing, that's called "branding." Do we want to be branded as being the same as everyone else, or do we want to be branded as something significantly *better*?

If our reputation is exceptional, meaning *not ordinary*, then we have earned the right to charge a fair fee that's labeled "uncustomary" by insurance carriers. In other words, if the value expectation exceeds the value a person puts on their money, then we have a viable business model that's based upon *our* philosophy, principles, values, skills, and judgment *as long as we are able to consistently deliver on the promise.* Suppose we are unable to create that kind of perception. In that case, the perception that what we do is exceptional from our target market's point of view, then we have a challenge ahead: We need to raise our game relative to skill set, comprehensive new patient experience, and marketing.

Dentists who, for the most part, avoid explanations in favor of helping patients think clearly are more likely to influence their behavior. The very fact that a dentist stops talking and attempts to get a patient to think for themselves conveys an interest in the patient and a desire for them to assume some self-control over their relationship. Almost without exception, patients welcome this challenge. As they think seriously about a plan of ultimately experience improved dental health.

~Robert F. Barkley, D.D.S.

Successful Preventive Dental Practices (1972)

Chapter 56
CoDiscovery & CoDiagnosis

Bob Barkley is credited with bringing the terms "CoDiscovery" and "CoDiagnosis" into our lexicon, and as a consequence, both are seen in many articles, books, and presentations. Rarely however is a distinction made between CoDiscovery and CoDiagnosis, so let's take a moment to clarify the differences:

CoDiscovery

CoDiscovery is best conceptualized as *learning with*. Bob Barkley intentionally structured his new patient experience to facilitate it— but learning with and about what? CoDiscovery was an experience for both himself and the new patient, wherein they'd learn more about what was going well and not-so-well their stomatognathic system:

- What is healthy?

- What is pathological?

- What is subjectively attractive to the person?

- What is unattractive to the person?

- What is functional?

- What is dysfunctional?

- What does the person know?

- What does the person understand?

- What is trending toward becoming a problem that has long-term implications?

- What is the patient experiencing on the emotional level as they learn more about themselves?

CoDiagnosis

CoDiagnosis, on the other hand, happens *after* CoDiscovery. It's the informed conversation focused on what the findings mean to the person on the physical, functional, and emotional levels. That discussion is carefully integrated into what the person thinks they'd like to do—and when. It has a purpose: "Success Planning." If a person isn't ready to participate in the design of a plan, or they aren't prepared to set goals for the future, then no definitive long-term plan is developed, and the patient is allowed time to think about what they want for themselves over time. If they are unable to do that, then a stabilization plan is created after permission is granted: "Would you like me to develop a plan that's intended to stop the disease processes and stabilize the current level of breakdown so you have more time to think about what you'd like to see happen long-term?"

Bob Barkley was so committed to his new patient process, that he wrote in his practice brochure, "While it is important that a dentist diagnose your mouth, it is far more important that YOU diagnose it. The extent to which you understand your mouth determines your ability to plan for your future."[96]

Ownership and Self-Responsibility

Ultimately, CoDiscovery and CoDiagnosis are about fostering ownership, self-responsibility, effective planning, and the establishment of healthy emotional boundaries. Stephen Covey called that "win-win." Bob liked to call it "the formation of a therapeutic alliance."

We come into the role of being a guide or as a teacher - as someone who provides a safe haven where the other person can be deeply seen and feels safe and secure. At other times, we are the expert on the notion of health and un-health, ease and disease. Yet, our patients are also experts in their own right, deeply knowledgeable in other domains. Our patients are certainly expert in being themselves - no one else shares this distinctive skill base. Even without a lot of self-awareness, our clients are still trying to be the best "them" they can be at that point in time. So, we come together as individuals, each with our own perspective and expertise, to find one another along this journey across time. Our job isn't to know everything, but rather to be the one who is present, attuned, and open to being in resonance with the way things are, and then to move forward together from there.

~Daniel J. Siegel, M.D. [97]

Chapter 57
Introduction to Bob Barkley's Three-Phase Adult Education

I am honored to have the opportunity to share how Bob Barkley used *Three Phase Adult Education*, as it dramatically changed my practice and many others. I recently interviewed Bob's clinical assistant, Helen Ruth, which helped me to better understand how and why Bob did things the way he did them, consequently, I've added commentary throughout the description below.

I recognize that dentistry has entered the digital age and therefore, many people might consider Bob's processes to be too antiquated, irrelevant, or time-consuming. Today, it's possible to examine and treat a patient without ever touching a plaster model or occlusal wax. It's also possible to complete an entire full-mouth reconstruction with the use of a digital articulator. However, as we move more and more into the digital realm, it's important to keep in mind that a significant part of human communication is non-verbal and that there's a lot of power in allowing a person to participate by literally "holding their mouth in their hands," (via physical master casts) and then be allowed the time to think while they are doing it.

Digital technology is a powerful communication tool; however, I recommend making a judicious marriage of the old with the new and not jettisoning too much of "the old" simply because there are now faster ways to do it. I decided to share *Three Phase Adult Education* toward the end of this book because I wanted you to first gain a deeper understanding of the neuroscience and psychology behind it. Understanding the *why* behind the *what* allows us to move forward while remaining true to the sophistication of Bob's work. This point is particularly relevant when we need to significantly expand a patient's understanding of their situation and create a more successful working relationship. A robust digital approach works well for those who are already "above the line" (people who are well-referred, already trust us, and already want what we have to offer), but we need to be careful as everyone learns in their own unique way, and what we think a person knows, understands, and values is often quite a bit different than what we assume.

Chapter 58
Three-Phase Adult Education

When a new *adult* patient was interested in joining Bob Barkley's practice, they were invited to join him for an informal meet-and-greet at the end of a clinical day (usually a Wednesday). At that time, the prospective patient would meet Bob in his private office, share a cup of coffee, and discuss their concerns, problems, and goals. The purpose of the meetings was to assess whether or not the two parties shared enough philosophical common ground that they were likely to be successful at establishing a long-term working relationship. The step was similar to how a person might interview an investment advisor: do they share your investment philosophy and understand your risk tolerance? Due to Bob's previous experiences and his success with his practice philosophy, he wasn't interested in attempting to start a new relationship without first verifying that the person was aware of the uniqueness of his practice and its benefits, from his point of view.

On that point, Bob said, *"People must realize that health is not a commodity to be purchased; it must be self-acquired. They must learn that the only things that dentistry can provide are improved comfort, function, and attractiveness."* Thus, without that kind of shared understanding, there was a high risk of miscommunication and frustration.

Bob said, *"We quite commonly get acquainted with patients' histories and vital statistics and spell out our office policies; yet rarely do we make a sincere effort to learn peoples' beliefs and attitudes and expose them to ours. Unless two people understand one another's frame of reference, communication is difficult or even distorted."*

It's also important to understand that most of Bob's new patients knew him socially on some level, due to the small size of the community. Thus, if you're not in a similar small-town situation, it's likely going to take a little more time to develop safe-feeling, trustworthy relationships. The author prefers to use pre-exam interviews combined with the continuation of that interview at the (next) preclinical visit. I do *not* use a Patient Care Coordinator for that role (notice there are several different ways to deploy these concepts *if* you understand the thinking behind them). Whether or not you use a Patient Care Coordinator is a decision you should make based on your interviewing skills, the strength of your care team, and the effectiveness of your ability to connect with new patients on more than a superficial level.

THREE PHASE ADULT EDUCATION

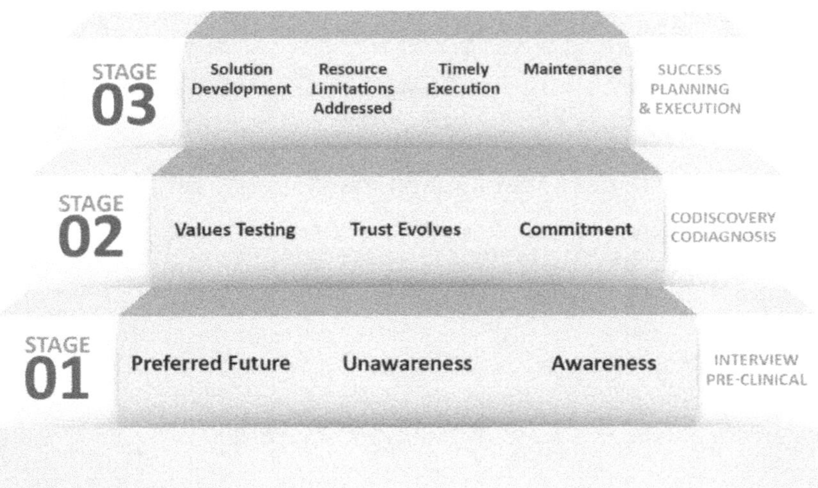

Outline of the Three-Phase Education Process

STAGE 1 — THE PRECLINICAL INTERVIEW

A. **Preferred Future** (The pre-clinical visit should allow the patient to consider and express their preferred long-term outcomes: the beginning of a preferred future)

B. Unawareness (Most patients enter partially or totally unaware of where they are health-wise, where they are headed, what that personally means, what they truly want, and what's possible)

C. Awareness (The Co-Discovery process leads to increased awareness and creates a strategic tension between where the person actually is and what they *say* they want for themselves long-term)

STAGE 2 — CoDISCOVERY & CoDIAGNOSIS

A. Values Testing: If the person's behaviors are not in alignment with their beliefs and preferred future, they must address the *disequilibria.*

B. Trust Evolves: The person starts to believe that you're the best resource to help resolve their problems and achieve their goals.

C. Commitment: The person commits to the pursuit of a preferred future, including the psychological process of owning the problem

STAGE 3 — SUCCESS PLANNING & EXECUTION

A. Solution Development: A *Success Plan* is co-developed.

B. Affordability Issues Addressed: Time, energy, and money issues are discussed and negotiated without compromising the quality of the plan.

C. Timely Execution: The plan is put into action.

D. Maintenance: The person remains committed to taking care of the successful outcome.

Note: The following is a narrative description of my interpretation of how Bob Barkley conducted *Three-Phase Adult Education*. It is not an exact duplication of how Bob described *TPAE* in his book *Successful Preventive Dental Practices*, to which I refer you if you'd like to see the original wording.

PHASE 1: Pre-Clinical Interview

In Bob's office, a *Patient Care Coordinator* (PCC) conducted the pre-clinical interview, strategically highlighting the primary reason the person called the office. Fifteen minutes was generally allowed for that aspect of the appointment which included a careful review of the patient's medical history. At that time, the PCC would work toward developing a trusting relationship. They would informally gather personal information, review the medical history with a particular emphasis on how the person felt about all of it, and then attempt to ascertain the level of the patient's orientation toward having a more whole-health philosophy.

The PCC would, at the appropriate time, share some of the unique qualities of the practice. For example, she would start to informally share a little bit about the practice philosophy – but only in very broad terms, and would simultaneously give the patient a customized practice brochure that contained an expanded version of it.

The PCC explained the practice is health and goal-oriented and that the purpose of the appointment was to *begin* gathering information associated with their current status, as well as organize the information in a way that allows them to learn more about where they were and what they might want to do going forward. As a part of the process, the PCC emphasized that an accurate diagnosis and a jointly created plan of action, was the most important thing they would ever do together, as the quality of everything happening after that point hinges on it. Meaning, that a well-designed plan leads them toward a "preferred future," whereas a poorly designed plan leads them toward mistakes, wasted time, undesired outcomes, and regrets.

The PCC explained that Bob felt treatment decisions should largely be driven by what the person wanted for themselves long-term, and therefore should be based on their goals.

The patient was informed:

The process would continue at the next visit after the model work, slide photography, and radiographs were prepared for review.

They would develop a plan together, and the patient would be in control of what they would do and when.

After completion of the evaluation and planning process, if the person doesn't feel that it was the most valuable time they have ever spent in a dental office, they are free to keep a copy of the x-rays, and they won't owe the practice anything for the cost of the examination, x-rays, and consultation.

The preclinical interview concept is based upon the belief that as the patient begins to align themselves with the practice philosophy, they'll also begin to accept members of the practice on a personal level and trust will naturally build over time.

Bob's approach allowed the new patient to *experience* the purpose of the practice, as well as perceive its value. Simultaneously, the patient experienced that the purpose of the practice wasn't simply to find problems and sell solutions. The "preclinical" step—the relationship development step—is vitally important, and should never be rushed. It's strategically designed to help each person think about dentistry and dental health in a more relevant and constructive fashion.

Why? Because trust, learning, and the development of creative solutions to problems are all right-brain functions that optimally occur when a person is relaxed, feels safe, and can see the value in solving/addressing the problems they are learning about.

Bob would reestablish a social connection and then weave into the conversation key points mentioned at the meet-and-greet visit. The conversation was unstructured and began wherever the person wanted to begin their story. After discussing issues that were top-of-mind, Bob used *reflective thinking* to take the patient back and re-live key memories associated with dentistry. Bob's goal was to help the person see how their problem(s) had evolved over time.

Bob accepted their story at face value, regardless of how distorted or inaccurate it was, and then transitioned into talking about the patient's preferred future. Finally, Bob redirected the conversation back to the present time and what the person was experiencing. The reflective thinking strategy was an attempt to prompt the patient to think about dentistry through a new mindset wherein the person could visualize how the past had influenced the present, and how the present was going to influence their future. The structure of the conversation created the opportunity for the patient to share what the new realizations meant to them. Were they feeling a sense of despair? Anxiety? Frightened? Concerned? Confident? Uncertain? Hopeful? Excited?

During Bob's preclinical interview time, he would discuss their dental history, such as decay frequency, the amount of dentistry they had previously experienced, how those appointments went, family patterns associated with dental problems, tooth loss, and so forth. He would probe issues such as: How they felt about losing their teeth and whether or not they felt it was going to be their fate. Do they see the same patterns they've experienced repeating in their children? What had the past five years been like for them in terms of dental needs? What was *their* philosophy toward dental health? Do they view dental health as something separate from their whole health, or do they view it as an integral part of it all? How much do they value dental health? What are their goals regarding dental health and the appearance of their teeth going forward? What are their primary concerns? Bob wanted to hear each person tell him how much they wanted to keep their natural teeth for the rest of their life – even if they weren't sure if it was a possibility.

Bob asked if they had any urgent issues that required immediate attention.* If there were none, Bob would tell the patient the purpose of the remaining part of their visit was to create study models (after showing them what study casts looked like) and films (after showing them what an FMX looked like) to build up value and relevance). The person was told that they would review the models and films together at the next visit, as well as discuss what the clinical findings revealed.

When a patient was experiencing an emergency (what Bob referred to as their "present preoccupation"), he would try and address it that day, or as quickly as possible. Additionally, he would make payment for that emergency service optional. His goal was to eliminate the "present preoccupation," a psychological barrier prohibiting the person from focusing their attention on long-term trends and their implications. Consequently, the CoDiscovery appointment was sometimes delayed until the urgency was addressed – at least on a provisional level.

That was why Bob had pre-examination "meet and greet" appointments *before* patients were scheduled for *Three Phase Examinations*. In that way, Bob strategically created an opportunity to explain how he preferred to work with people and why. And at that point, a person was able to opt-out if they felt like they weren't interested in engaging in a more health-centered approach to dentistry.

Note: *Bob emphasized that he didn't want his care team to try and explain the three-stage adult education process to patients in advance, and to particularly avoid doing so over the phone, as it was too easily misinterpreted.* <u>Bob felt that the value of the comprehensive examination and the CoDiscovery process was best promoted in-person.</u>

Bob Barkley's practice was primarily a restorative practice, and it included people who were either restored or who were moving toward full restoration. **Note:** *Bob would not take a patient through the* Three Stage Adult Education *process when they only had minimal needs and were already in a state of independent health. Additionally, he would not take people through the process unless they showed interest in learning more about their situation.*

PHASE 2: CoDiscovery/CoDiagnosis

The second visit began in the treatment room with Bob's clinical assistant handing unmounted study models to the patient, inviting them to "take a look," and then informing the person that Bob would be with them shortly. She would exit the room for the purpose of strategically allowing the person time to become more familiar with the condition of their teeth. Bob believed that mounting models initially on an articulator caused a "loss of spontaneity," but would later put them on an articulator to demonstrate occlusal interferences and guidance issues.

After a few minutes, Bob entered the examination room, asked the patient what they were looking at and thinking about. That is where the discussion would begin, and from there, he would take the patient through a carefully sequenced learning process:

1. First, the assistant would ask, **"Are there any missing teeth?"** If so, Bob would point them out on the models and then ask the patient (when relevant), "Have you ever considered replacing them?"

2. The assistant would then ask, **"Position of remaining teeth?"** Bob would ask, "Do you know what happens when your teeth drift like this?"—while using the model to point to the specific example.

3. The assistant would ask, **"Any disfigurement of the anterior teeth?"** Bob, using the models to demonstrate, would ask, "Do you see how these teeth fit together? Were you aware that this is happening?"—Bob would then point out where facets, etc.

Note: We were all trained to perform static examinations that identify what is wrong with a mouth/dentition. The intention here is to create a *dynamic examination* wherein the patient can experience: "Is this me? Is that what's really happening to me?"

1. The assistant would ask, **"Any evidence of bruxism?"** If present, Bob would point out the attrition and help the patient to visualize its long-term implications.

2. The assistant would ask, **"Are there any pseudo pockets** (due to inclined teeth)?" If, present Bob would explain.

3. The assistant would ask, **"Is there any loss of papilla?** And then Bob would ask, "Did you know that your gums are receding over here? Do you know why having gums between your teeth is so important?"

4. The assistant would ask, **"Any generalized recession?"** Bob would say, "Have you noticed…"

Note: Creating dissatisfaction with the present circumstance is key to catalyzing change. Bob Barkley called this "catalyzing a change in attitude toward the problem," and that's centrally what the CoDiscovery process was intended to do—to strategically create some tension in the mind of the person between where they thought they were health-wise, and then juxtapose it against where the person *learns* they are (not just told).

1. The assistant would ask, **"Any evidence of erosion?"** If present, Bob would talk about the various ways erosion can occur. He also discussed how tooth sensitivity was often linked to the abrasives present in toothpastes.

2. The assistant would ask, **"Any broken fillings?"** If there were any broken fillings, Bob would then ask, "Do you have any idea why your fillings are broken?" and "Has this been a common problem for you?" Bob would use those questions to segue into stating his philosophy toward restoration: "We would like to get you to a place where when the time comes to restore your teeth, we'll do it in the very best way possible, and therefore we will be able to significantly reduce the chance that these teeth will ever need to be repaired again. How do you feel about using that type of approach? We can use materials that look nice *and* are largely unbreakable."

Note: Bob would intentionally avoid over-explanations and try to keep things on the simplest and most appropriate level of understanding, except for those patients who asked for more details.

1. The assistant would ask, **"How are the margins of the old fillings?"** Bob would explain, "When the margin of a filling is failing because the tooth broke adjacent to it, then we can understand why that happened. When a margin is failing because of a seal issue, it may be a process error on the part of the dentist."

2. The assistant would ask, **"Any occlusal interferences?"** Bob would mount the models on an articulator and then demonstrate guidance, initial points of contact, balancing interferences, etc., and then he would associate the observations with an accelerated breakdown of dentistry or teeth.

Note: Bob viewed this step as a "dress rehearsal" for what they would soon be doing in the mouth. He was intentionally building awareness and familiarity with important concepts that he wanted the patient to learn more about, so that they would be able to make better decisions later during the treatment planning process. He would then check the occlusion in the mouth by marking the initial contact point as well as excursive contacts in the posterior, where there was potential for future cusp fractures and tooth cracking.

1. The assistant would ask, **"Are there any potential cusp fracture areas?"** These would be pointed out to the patient on the mounted models. All the likely future cusp fracture sites were noted. In that way, the patient could *see* the association between how their bite functioned and how teeth could break.

Note: This is powerful learning, and the more skillful we become at facilitating it, the more the patient will learn. The more the patient learns, the more likely they are to say "yes" to an optimal treatment plan.

1. The assistant would ask, **"Are there any food impaction sites or unmanageable bacterial traps?"** Bob would then ask, "When you are out to eat, does food ever get caught between

your teeth and you wish you had some way to get it out of there?"

Note: Bob found that if you simply ask, "Do you have any places where food catches between your teeth?" the question "too often elicited a negative response even when there were obvious contact-related issues."

1. **Next, the radiographs were reviewed**:

    a. Prevalence of fillings?

    b. Overhanging margins?

    c. Recurrent cavities?

    d. New cavities? – he would point them out to the patient, but would not finalize charting.

    e. Periapical infections?

    f. Widened periodontal ligaments?

    g. Any un-erupted teeth?

    h. General appearance of the supporting bone?

As the assistant asked the questions, Bob would put an X-ray light box in his lap while sitting beside the patient and answer the questions that were posed by his assistant.

Note: *Bob would intentionally not look at the X-rays or the models in advance of the CoDiscovery examination,* so that he would learn at the same time as the patient. This was a clever adjustment that Bob made to stop himself from talking too much and presenting solutions to problems too quickly. Since Bob was such a good and enthusiastic salesman of dental treatment, the approach forced Bob into a situation where he couldn't easily get ahead of the patient's understanding, and then wander off into elaborate explanations that confused the patient, or caused the person to agree before they understood their situation well enough to be able to take full ownership. In short, Bob wanted the whole experience to be spontaneous: "I am not smart enough to pull that off if I have seen things beforehand. And I don't feel honest about it if I have seen it before, because *I am honestly wanting to learn with them*. I am not a good enough teacher to teach, but if I can get them to learn with me, I will not have to teach them."

3. The assistant would ask, **"Any bone loss?"** When present, Bob would describe all bone loss in percentages: "Yes, we have about 30% bone loss over here…" And then Bob would say, "Did you know that your jawbone is going away? This allowed Bob the opportunity to show where the bone level was located and where it had been historically. He would then ask, "Do you know why your bone goes away like that?" And the patient would rarely know, but it opened up the conversation so that Bob could explain possible causes.

Note: Bob made the information *relevant* before presenting it.

1. The assistant would ask, **"Any angular bone loss?"** Bob would say, "Do you know why that's happening? It's because that tooth is getting over-loaded, and it will cause you to possibly lose the tooth over time. We would like all your teeth to hit evenly at the same time when you bite down and not bump into each other when you chew. Does that sound like a good thing to you?"

Note this key point: As you proceed through this process, you need to identify as many positive things to comment on as you can find, so the person does not feel overwhelmed by all of the negative findings, and you avoid building up a doomsday scenario in their mind. You want the patient to exit the CoDiscovery process feeling hopeful and that you are the most careful, concerned, and thorough dentist they have ever met. Try to make comments such as, "I have patients who would give anything to have the kind of bone you have around your teeth," "This is a really good thing," or "Even though you have had a lot of fillings in the past, most of your teeth are still structurally sound, and I do not see any reason that you will lose any more of your teeth in the future."

1. The assistant would ask, **"What is the condition of the temporomandibular joints?"** Bob would ask the patient to close their ear canals with their fingers and then open and close their mouth, and ask, "Do you hear anything?" And if there was a click, he would say, "Does that always happen? How long has that been going on?" He would then try to correlate the sound to something happening with the occlusion, "That's on the same side your teeth hit heavy, isn't it? It might be that your bite being off caused the jaw joint disc to break down, so the jaw clicking is a symptom of the bite being off."

2. The assistant would say, **"Oral cancer inspection,"** and Bob would comment on relevant findings.

The assistant would say, **"Periodontal examination,"** and a periodontal charting was made, including mobility and recession. Bob would ask questions about how much their gums bled and when. Next, he would talk about how gingival bleeding was an indication that the "skin on their gums was damaged" and the damage was allowing bacteria to enter their bloodstream with the potential to cause infection and inflammation. Bob would identify areas of heavy plaque accumulation and make a point of letting the patient know that it wasn't just something left over from eating. At that point, he would take a plaque sample and put it under his phase contrast microscope and let the patient see the bacterial colonies. He also noted the pattern of calculus accumulation and would ask the patient how quickly it tended to build up.

Note: Bob would try to keep the learning on a basic level as well as get patients with decay and periodontal problems to accept that they had an active disease process, and that their problems weren't happening just because they have "bad teeth." He would say, "We know that the bacteria, some of which are streptococcus, can enter the bloodstream and cause systemic problems with the heart, pregnancy, and other issues." Bob used a phase contrast microscope to reinforce these concepts and to reinforce that the mouth is a biosystem that's either in or out of balance.

1. The assistant would ask, **"Any chronic problems with bad breath?"** Bob would respond to the possible causes, with the most common being periodontal disease.

2. The assistant would ask, **"Are there any unmanageable teeth?"** Bob would then plan for their removal when appropriate ASAP while telling the patient, "After these teeth are removed, we do not want to remove any more teeth over your lifetime."

3. The assistant would ask, **"Dental decay? Active, very active, limited, or very limited?"** Bob would comment on the biosystem being out of balance, if decay was present.

4. The assistant would ask, **"Are there any cracked teeth?"** Bob would call out the findings.

5. The assistant would ask, **"Sleep quality history? Snoring?"** Bob would talk about the importance of restful sleep and the need to keep weight within a healthy range.

6. The assistant would ask, **"What is the general appearance of the teeth?"** Bob would inquire how the patient felt about the appearance of their teeth, and discuss what they would like improve – if anything.

7. The assistant would ask, **"What is the general appearance of the mouth?"** This question was intended to transition the conversation over to an overview of the previous findings and the comments made by the patient. Bob would ask how the patient felt about the appearance of their teeth and smile, as well as how much of a priority it was to them to improve their condition.

Important Note on Fees: No fees were charged for models or X-rays. The only fee Bob charged was a fee for his diagnosis and plan. The fee for the diagnosis was only presented when the patient was interested and asked him to develop a comprehensive plan. Otherwise, the patient would not enter the practice, or only a *Phase One Plan* was presented and the development of a comprehensive plan was delayed until disease stabilization was achieved, or the patient's financial "readiness" improved.

About 1 out of 10 people (in non-fluoridated Macomb in 1970) had minimal needs. A third visit wasn't necessary for those patients, and they were scheduled for appropriate treatment after the second appointment. The others, who indicated that they were interested in having Bob create a comprehensive plan, were scheduled for a third appointment to discuss the plan.

PHASE 3: Success Planning

At the end of Phase 2, and after the patient had departed, Bob would dictate his findings as well as create an optimal comprehensive treatment plan broken down into phases. It included all significant findings, trends, what's possible correction-wise, and what that would mean long-term relative to what the patient said they wanted to see happen. An order of treatment was recommended, including disease control work when appropriate. Bob stated that 50% of his new patients did not need disease control.

At the third appointment, Bob had the patient read his written report in the reception area, and then would review the contents of the report in his consultation room. He would go through the report paragraph by paragraph and encourage the patient to ask questions.

In discussing the plan, Bob would mention the limitations associated with treatment, such as the possibility of pulp deaths in the future and the implications of bruxism on tooth/restoration longevity. He would explain that the plan involved a lot of things to consider, as well as a solid commitment to follow through with all of it to be successful. He also told the patient that he would understand if they were not ready to do everything all at one time, and if that was the case, they were welcome to stay in the practice.

The dictated report was written in a way that it was easy to understand, used lay terminology, and included feelings about the patient's future, with and without treatment. By allowing the patient to read the report in the patient lounge before discussing it, the patient had more time to think about it and to prepare questions. After managing the patient's questions and concerns, Bob quoted the fee for each phase only when the patient indicated that they were ready to proceed. Then Bob would ask, "What do you think?" Sometimes a negotiation process ensued for the purpose of keeping the desired plan within the patient's budget or to match it to their scheduling limitations.

The written treatment plan represented a long-range blueprint of what needed to happen over time to achieve optimal health, function, and esthetics. Bob wrote:

This written copy is not a motivational piece, although it does put it all together in a concise, orderly fashion. Hopes, desires, fears and dislikes are dealt with, and a sequence of goals is established that allows for one successful experience after another. It, in essence, is a program that allows the patient to look into his dental future with a reasonable level of confidence.

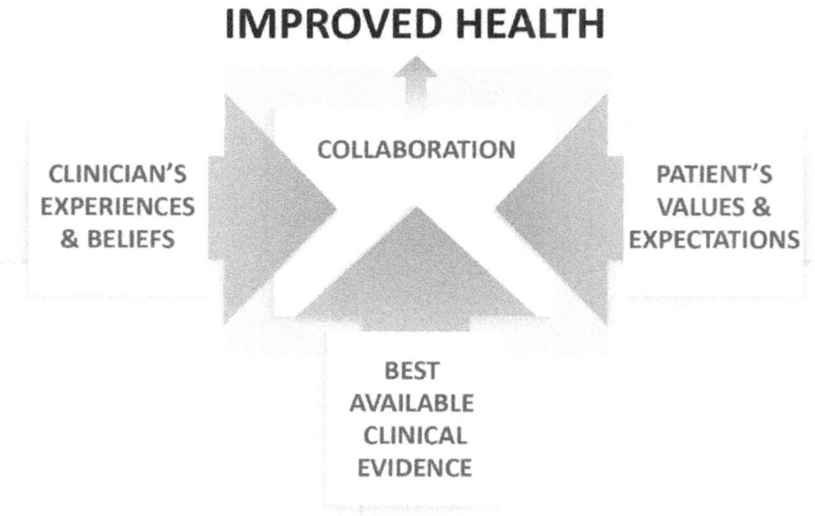

My Experience with this Process

I have successfully integrated Three-Phase Adult Education into my practice via some additions and modifications. Due to the incredible educational power of digital photography, I review digital photographs captured at the first visit *at the beginning of the second* visit (set up in a Powerpoint® file format), *before we proceed into the CoDiscovery examination.* The patient is seated in my conference room, and we review the photographs and radiographs together—during which, I speak only in general terms and offer no solutions: "Notice the cracks in this tooth—that's something we'll want to take a look at when we go back and complete the examination." Those types of general comments open the door for the patient to make statements like "I had no idea my teeth were in this condition." To which I'll respond, "It might look bad, but I've seen much worse situations. Let's gather more information before we make a decision about what we want to do about it" (Notice: I am using "we" and not "I"). So, I do things in that order—review photographs and radiographs with the person sitting next to me, for the purpose of creating more relevance to clinical findings that will soon be "discovered" (again) during the CoDiscovery examination.

Another example: The patient will comment on an area of obvious clinical recession in the photographs. In response, I'll show them the corresponding area in a radiograph that demonstrates bone loss –the *reason* the tissue receded. Or, I'll point out an area of inflamed soft tissue and correlate the clinical sign to calculus in a radiograph or to radiographic bone loss. As a result, when we proceed into the physical aspect of the CoDiscovery examination (we are in an examination room at that point), the findings are much more relevant to the person because their mind has been *primed,* and I can say things like, "Do you remember the area in the photograph where your gums were receded? Well, this is the same area in your mouth. Notice how easily it bleeds…notice how my measuring instrument goes down deeper right here—that's where the bone was missing on the x-ray." Teaching in this strategic fashion allows me to emphasize important learning points 3-5 times: 1) On a photograph, 2) On a radiograph, 3) On mounted study casts, 4) In their mouth (or perhaps) 5) On a CBCT. *Doing things in that fashion significantly increases memory retention, relevance, engagement, concern, and it helps turn a new belief into a commitment to take action!*

We do not take study models on every patient, although we do in most cases, as my practice is generally adult restorative/TMD/ Sleep. So, mounted study casts are a fairly regular part of our routine, and my facility is set up nicely to organize and store study models. We also use our iTero scanner to create digital records. Additionally, we use a phase contrast microscope to look at plaque samples *with* patients who have gingival bleeding and/or evidence of active periodontal disease at the first visit. That's a powerful form of CoDiscovery as well. The intention is to facilitate their understanding of bacterial, yeast, and/or parasitic infections and that the bleeding is associated with more than just inadequate brushing or flossing. PCR or genomic periodontal pocket testing periodontal pocket testing is used when the plaque sample merits that step. The test results are discussed at the second visit and coordinated with treatment planning. Additionally, I use an online STOP-Bang sleep apnea assessment that's set up on an iPad during the first appointment interview, with the findings revisited at the second appointment when relevant. I will use a take-home sleep apnea screening device between the first and second visits when that's appropriate as well. So, my clinical examination is much more slanted toward screening for sleep issues than Bob's was, as it includes a Mallampati score, measurement of maxillary arch width, tongue-tie assessment, tonsils, and so forth.

Lastly, it's important to understand that Three Phase Adult Education must be iterative and personalized. In many cases, depending on the complexity of the situation, the amount of specialist support required, and the cooperation and commitment of the patient, it might take more than three appointments to get to a place where a "success plan" can be finalized. The author has had multiple cases that have taken years to complete, as the patient required TM joint surgery, orthognathic surgery, orthodontics, etc., *before* the final restorative phase was definitively planned. In those cases, only estimates could be developed and the patient had to be comfortable with some of the ambiguity associated with time and cost. In other words, their commitment to their preferred outcome had to be stronger than their need to have a guaranteed timeline or a total case fee on the front end of a long, complex, iterative rehabilitative process. These situations require a lot of trust, and that's why engaging the patient on a deeper level is critically important. Without a person's understanding of the bigger picture, it becomes easy for unanticipated bumps in the road to destroy a restorative process mid-stream.

217

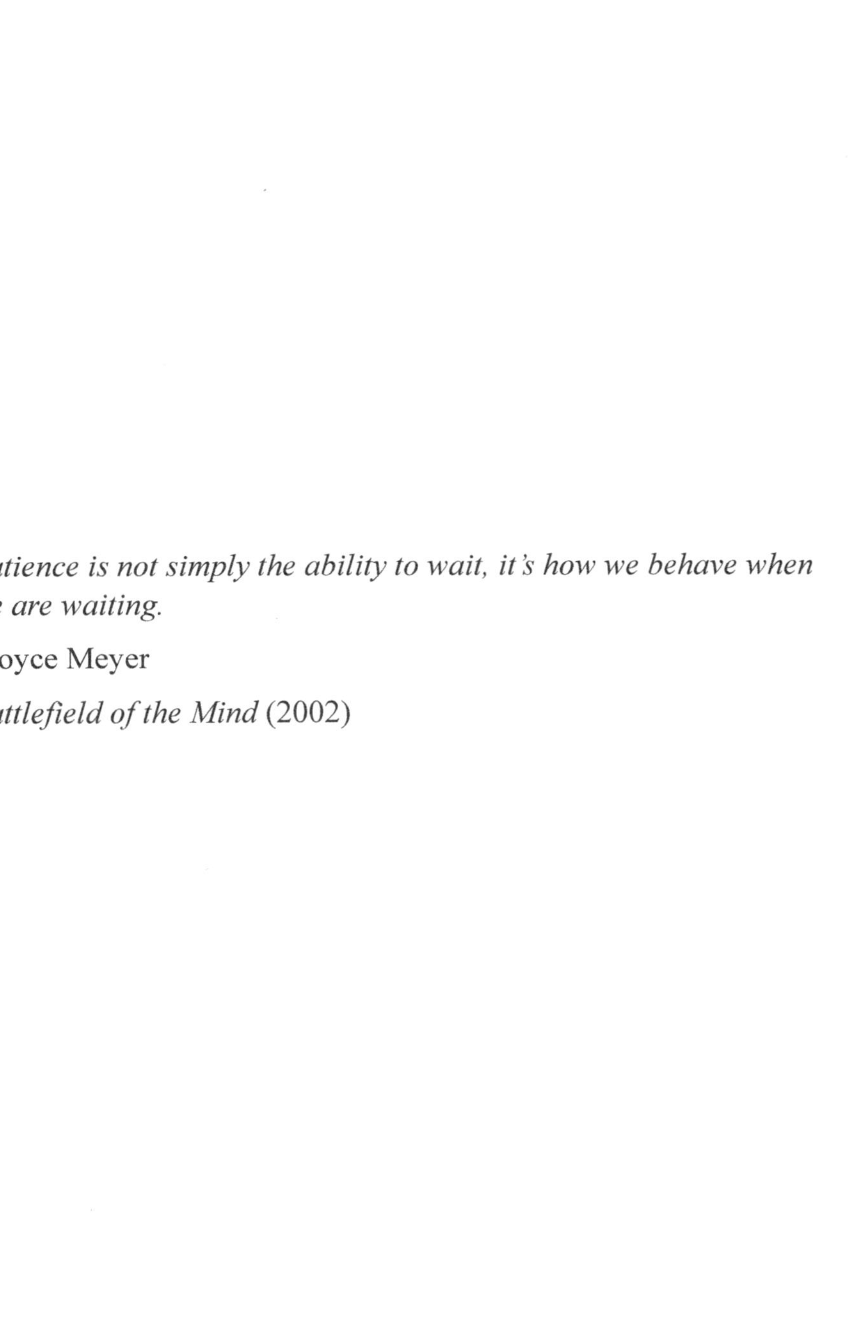

Patience is not simply the ability to wait, it's how we behave when we are waiting.

~Joyce Meyer

Battlefield of the Mind (2002)

Chapter 59
The Future

Only a few months before his untimely death, Bob Barkley wrote a thoughtful essay titled, *On Becoming a Humanistic Dentist*. At that point, Bob had been teaching his preventive-restorative philosophy for over ten years, yet only a small percentage of dentists had successfully implemented the concepts. Reflectively he said, *"Their dreams have not yet been realized because they approached a philosophical conversion of themselves in a mechanical way. They simply added new techniques and tactics without adequately redefining their roles, or they simply added new techniques and tactics without adequately examining their values and beliefs about dentistry and their relationships with people."*

As discussed in previous chapters, successful health-centered practices require a different mindset focused on a relationship-driven, health-centered mission. Prevention must precede repair and restoration, or it will likely fail; hence, the former should rarely precede the latter, yet most dentists do it out of frustration and financial need. That outcome aligns well with the opening passage of Dickens' *A Tale of Two Cities*, "It was the best of times; it was the worst of times," as our profession has never been better at diagnosing, correcting, and repairing, yet the National Institute of Dental and Craniofacial Research tells us, "Dental caries remains the most prevalent chronic disease in both children and adults,"[98] and roughly 42 percent of all dentate U.S. adults 30 years of age or older have periodontitis.[99] If we add the 22 million Americans suffering with obstructive sleep apnea,[100] and the obesity, diabetes, autism, and ADHD epidemics, we have a massive health crisis nested within a medical system that's frequently unable to understand or eliminate root causes frequently related to dysfunctions of the stomatognathic system, nasopharyngeal system, and/or the oral microbiome.

Our current situation: ubiquitous CBCT machines, high-resolution radiography, scanners, lasers, computer modeling, milling machines, sophisticated restorative materials, dental "insurance," antibiotics, disinfectants, biocides, "same-day dentistry" and doc-in-a-boxes servicing people who are often becoming *less* healthy over time. Many observers call it *sickness-centered care,* wherein dentists have been downgraded to "provider" status, and patients are marketed to sheep for cures that often fail to deliver on the implied promises—or worse."[101]

To quote Bob Barkley in *Successful Preventive Dental Practices:* *"A difficult dilemma confronts us when we consider the topic of will, discussion, and responsibility in relation to health. The dilemma is that the new scientific discoveries and techniques for curing people, within the physical and psychological spheres, tend to make them the object of cure, whereas health, in its deeper and authentic sense, can come only with the growth of the sense of responsibility on the part of the patient. "* And that requires a much more effective doctor-patient relationship that combines each person's concerns, problems, and goals with multi-disciplinary leadership. Put another way, we can't get there just by leveraging more technology, scaling up, and improving workflow. Hence, success is highly related to our ability to know our patients in more significant ways, help them to learn more about oral-systemic connections, and lead them toward sustainable health by dealing with the root-cause issues; we need to move well beyond mechanical and pharmacological approaches if we want to treat complex biological, behavioral, and developmental problems in a successful fashion.

Throughout this book, I hope I have made it clear that what patients *act like they want* frequently isn't what they truly desire. *What most people want is a feeling,* they want to *feel* healthy and satisfied with how their teeth look. They want restful sleep and to *feel* refreshed in the morning. They want to *feel* comfortable, safe, heard, and valued, and they want to spend money only on things they *feel* are important, relevant, and timely.

How can we achieve these outcomes on a daily basis?—Through what Bob Barkley called "attitudinal development," wherein:

The dentist must help guide the patient's thinking or, in most cases, introspection (values clarification and long-term planning) will not occur. This is true because, without guidance, many dental patients think of dentistry only in terms of cost (time, energy, money) rather than what they'd really like for their mouths. In dentistry, such inverted thinking often leads to senseless extractions or inferior repairs. [102]

Getting people to want what they need requires leadership and learning within a health-centered relationship—a one-on-one game that isn't always immediately rewarded, convenient, or efficient.

Human relationships are unpredictable, messy, and inefficient, yet, when we assume a developmental mindset, we see these complex situations through a different set of eyes, revealing tremendous opportunities if we adjust our practice systems.

There is no question that consolidation, industrialization, and micromanagement will continue to spread across the dental profession at an increasing rate, yet that doesn't need to be your fate. You have a choice, as there is a different pathway, and the good news is that many who are currently traveling that pathway are showing us how to follow. From their perspective, dentists are in the best position of all the health professions to positively change the health trajectories of millions of people due to their familiarity with the stomatognathic system, nasopharyngeal system, and oral microbiome. Additionally, we are in an ideal position to develop deeper, more meaningful and effective health-centered working relationships.

The following graphic illustrates this point.

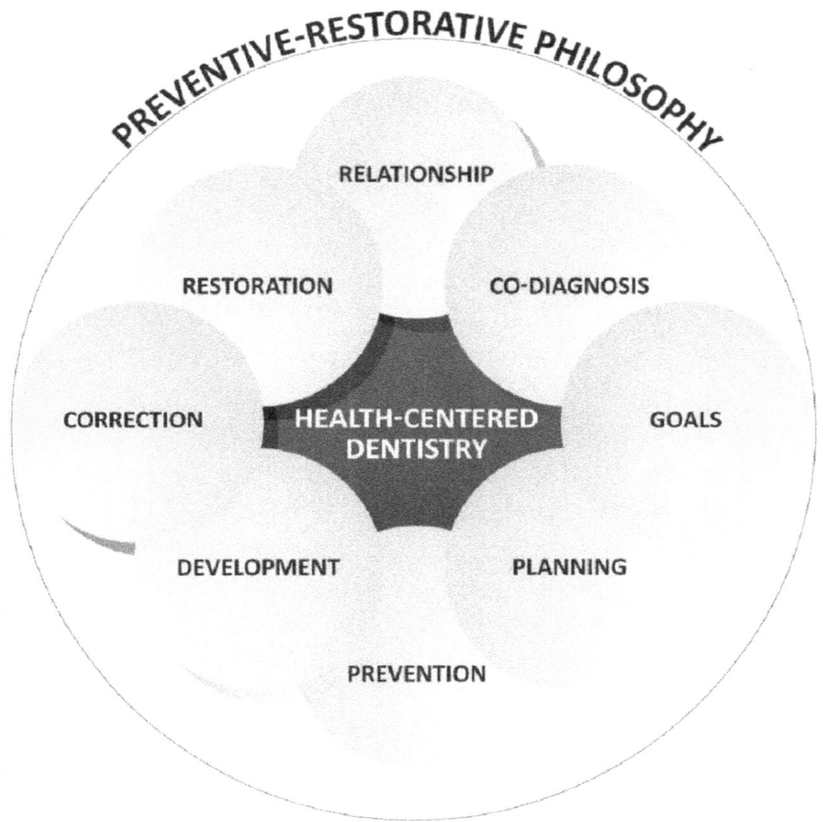

Relationship

Health-centered dentistry begins with a healthy, open, honest, trustworthy relationship between the dentist and patient, as without this type of relationship, we function independently as best, and co-dependently at worst. When a person has complex problems that require significant outside assistance to resolve them, a successful *inter*dependent relationship becomes absolutely essential.

Co-diagnosis

Successful CoDiagnosis is the *outcome* of a safe, open, honest, learning-oriented, collaborative relationship.

Goals

Mutually agreed-upon goals can only be established when all participants in the relationship understand the value behind what needs to be accomplished, how, when, and why. Hence, health-centered goals can only be developed and executed when a successful, interdependent, collaborative relationship has been established and nurtured.

Planning

Effective planning becomes possible when clear, mutually agreed-upon goals have been established, some of which require interdisciplinary input and participation. For instance, a successful plan for an adult patient with growth and development problems in combination with occlusal dysfunction and disordered breathing/sleep apnea often requires a treatment team of dental specialists, medical specialists, a restorative dentist, and others working in a highly coordinated fashion.

Prevention

Commonly, some aspects of a patient's problem set involve their decisions and behavior, which are contributing to the severity of their problems, such as diet, hygiene habits, smoking, or other co-factors. Oftentimes, one issue feeds on others, such as a dry mouth due to allergy-driven mouth-breathing combined with a habit of high-carbohydrate snack consumption before bedtime. Until all causative factors are addressed, the disease state(s) cannot be stabilized or eliminated, which puts all repair and restorative attempts at a high risk of failure.

Development

Development can take on physical, psychological, and even spiritual forms. Some examples: 1) The deployment of interceptive orofacial growth and development strategies before the age of three so that a child will develop a strong tongue, proper dental arch form and lip seal, which then facilitate the development of optimal adult airway formation. 2) Stabilization of temporomandibular joints via occlusal orthotic therapy. 3) Pre-restorative arch form development via orthodontics. 4) Dental arch form development via bone grafting, surgically facilitated rapid orthodontic movement, or other procedures. 5) A shift in a patient's attitude toward their problem, via a growing understanding that they have more influence over their health outcome than previously assumed. 6) The realization that the body has amazing healing capacities if we simply give it the opportunity to reestablish homeostasis.

Correction

Correction can be as simple as an equilibration, or as complex as a full-mouth rehabilitation following TM joint therapy, periodontal treatment, and orthognathic surgery. Regardless, correction should be made in support of the attainment of shared long-term goals.

Restoration

Restoration in dentistry can be defined *as the act of restoring to a former condition, or the replacement of something lost or never properly developed.* Restoration can include the physical, functional, physiological, and psychological. Optimal restoration is only possible within the context of a truly helping relationship, clear-headed and mutually valued goals, careful execution, and follow-through. In many cases, successful restoration occurs after careful correction and the body's systems have been given a chance to accommodate and adapt.

Philosophy

A practice philosophy is the over-arching "WHY," hence none of the preceding steps can be well-coordinated and well-executed without it being so clear in the mind of the leader that it's consistently communicated to the treatment team and patients on both verbal and non-verbal levels. In the case of the author's practice, our Philosophy Statement reads:

Our Philosophy

To provide those we are privileged to serve with the very finest dental health advice and care through collaborative, health-centered relationships. These relationships shall be founded on integrity, trust, and our unwavering commitment to help others discover and obtain their desired long-term health future.

Chapter 60
More Thought Leaders Showing Us the Way

DeWitt Wilkerson advocates for "Integrative Dental Medicine," which includes "the 4 B's":

1. A properly functioning **B**ite, including its relationship to the entire masticatory system.

2. Appropriate management of **B**acteria and other oral pathogens to create a stable, healthy oral microbiome.

3. Appropriate **B**reathing capacity, so the body can optimally rest, digest, and heal.

4. Reduction of systemic inflammation in the **B**ody through proper nutrition, physical activity, and stress reduction.

DeWitt embraces a holistic perspective that views the stomatognathic system resting within a much bigger, divinely inspired whole-body system. On that topic, DeWitt authored an exceptional guidebook titled *The Shift, The Dramatic Movement Toward Health Centered Dentistry.* DeWitt can be contacted at www.estheticintegrativedentistry.com

***

Tom Larkin helps dentists to develop what he calls, "Biological, Health-oriented, Dental Practices," which are, according to Tom, "the largest emerging market opportunity in modern history." On that topic, Tom said:

There is a small group of individuals working within dentistry today, creating an exciting new category of change. These dentists and team members have learned that by focusing on the education and clinical protocols that connect oral health to overall health, they can impact patients' lives on a level never dreamed of before. They are attaining purpose-driven happiness and improved career satisfaction. And they are separating themselves from the commoditized masses. They look upon the difficulties facing dentistry today as a challenge and opportunity for disruption. The doom and gloom of the DSO next door simply isn't on their radar.

Tom collaborated with Sue Rusalen to create *The Larkin Protocol*, a revolutionary approach that brings together the latest technology, tools, and training to identify problems with more speed and precision. The protocol includes the integration of video phase contrast microscopes as a form of Codiscovery, along with periodontal pocket testing, and advanced treatment strategies including ozonated water, lasers, nutrition counseling, and pre-biotics. For more information, visit www.powhygiene.com and tomlarkin.com

***

Sandra Kahn is an orthodontist and dentofacial orthopedics practitioner in Redwood City, CA. She received her graduate orthodontic training at the University of the Pacific, where she served on the craniofacial teams at UCSF and Stanford. Additionally, she completed graduate work at UC Berkeley, in human craniofacial growth and development. Sandra is the author of *Let's Face It – a guide to your child's optimal health, facial and dental development,* in addition to creating *Forwardontics*, a treatment philosophy platform that "focuses on the face and the causes of malocclusion." Additionally, she is the creator of the GOpex™ program (Good Oral Hygiene Posture Exercises), and the Up-Locker Vacuum Activator,™ an oral muscle training system. You can learn more about Sandra's work at www.forwardontics.com

***

Emily Stein attended the University of Iowa, where she earned her degree in microbiology. Next, she studied how bacteria behave, consume, and socialize for survival in every known environment at UC Berkeley, where she earned her PhD. Emily completed a Post-Doctorate Fellowship in Immunology and Rheumatology at Stanford where she deepened her understanding of the relationship between bacteria, inflammatory responses, and autoimmune disorders. Currently she is founder and Technical CEO of *Primal Health, LLC, a* company focused on the discovery, development, and marketing of *pre-biotics*, micronutrients used to influence the behavior of bacteria within various microbiomes. Emily's particular interest is the microbiome of the oral cavity – the second most diverse microbial compartment in the body, within which dental caries, gingivitis, and periodontal disease originate and facilitate the propagation of pathogens throughout the body via the bloodstream and swallowing. Emily studied the polymicrobial communities of the mouth, including all of their disbiotic states. From there, she developed and patented pre-biotics that negatively influence oral pathogens as they attempt to colonize and propagate throughout the oral biofilm. More specifically, Emily discovered how to suppress the populations of S. mutans, C. gingivalis, Treponema denticola, Tannerella forsythia, Porphyromonas gingivalis and others. Additionally, she promotes amino acid catabolism instead of carbohydrate catabolism, which minimizes acid production along with other destructive metabolites. The net result is the establishment of a helpful, symbiotic biofilm wherein pathogens are managed down to non-threatening levels, and a higher pH level is created that supports recalcification and resistance. A clinical study in collaboration with the Benjamin Rose Institute on Aging demonstrated a 78% reduction in plaque and no gingival bleeding in the test group taking PTx800 lozenges three times a day compared to placebo.[103] Read that again, because it's game-changing. Nurturing helpful bacteria and disrupting pathogenic bacteria's catabolism is what creates the difference between disease and health. Emily's ideas are safe, sustainable, and perhaps best of all, bacteria cannot adapt or become resistant to them like they can to xylitol, antibiotics, and other anit-microbials. Her products are available at dailydentalcares.com

***

David McCarty is a 1997 graduate of Duke University School of Medicine, completed his Internal Medicine Residency in 2000, and his Fellowship in Sleep Medicine at LSU in 2007. David is currently the Chief Medical Officer at Rebis Health where he collaborates with dentists and other specialists to bring a comprehensive approach to the practice of Sleep Medicine via his patient-centered philosophy. He is the author of *Ockham's Razor: Redefining Problem-solving in Clinical Sleep Medicine, Empowered Sleep Apnea*, and the host of the *Empowered Sleep Apnea Podcast*. David can be contacted at dave@EmpoweredSleepApnea.com

***

Roger Price is an Integrative Health and Functional Airway Specialist at Breathing Well Pty Limited. He is passionate about discovering new ways to move beyond the current "symptoms-treatment" model that "does little, if nothing, to identify the source of the health issue, and only masks the symptoms." Roger is a pharmacist by training who went on to study integrative medicine at the University of Southern Queensland, Australia, in addition to working with British dentist John Flutter and American dentist Barry Raphael, studying early intervention in children. Roger believes that a "seismic change" is necessary to address the pandemic of disrupted sleep. "We have to change the way that the delivery of solutions is presented," he says. "Today, by and large, with oral appliance therapy, the signing of the patient, the informed consent and the payment (usually up front) of several thousand dollars is the starting point. Only after that has happened and the appliance treatment has started, do the associated problems start to show themselves, and very often in the form of 'nothing is happening the way I thought it would'. If the dentist doesn't understand the postural, structural, behavioral, biochemical, nutritional and emotional implications associated with the lack of progress, then the temptation is to 'crank things up' to see if that will drive the change. … We have to find a way to vastly enlarge the pool of available experts with which people who have these complex issues can consult." Roger is currently working on the creation of a network of coordinated experts and treatment facilitators across medicine, dentistry, and other specialties to bridge that gap. Roger can be reached at admin@breathing-well.com

***

Rebecca Bockow is a graduate of The University of Washington School of Dentistry, after which she received her Master's Degree in Oral Biology with Board Certification in both orthodontics and periodontics from The University of Pennsylvania School of Dental Medicine. She says**,** *"Dentistry is my passion. I am particularly interested in understanding how and why malocclusions develop, as well as how to orthodontically set up the foundation for the restorative dentist and the interdisciplinary team."* Dr. Bockow lectures internationally on topics ranging from interdisciplinary treatment planning to airway and sleep disorders, skeletal growth and development, and corticotomy-facilitated orthodontic therapy. Dr. Bockow maintains a private practice, *Inspired Orthodontics*, in the Seattle area that's limited to orthodontics and periodontics, and is a Spear Education Resident Faculty member. You can learn more about Rebecca's work and practice at inspireortho.com

***

Stephen Carstensen, is a graduate of Baylor College of Dentistry and serves as a consultant to the American Dental Association for sleep-related breathing disorders. Additionally, he practices clinically at Premier Sleep Associates in Bellevue, Washington. A lifelong educator, Dr. Carstensen is currently the sleep education director for both Pankey Institute and Spear Education. He is also certified by the American Board of Dental Sleep Medicine, as well

229

as PastPresident. Steve can be reached at stevec@medmarkmedia.com

***

Michael Edwards, Director of the Schuster Center, leads workshops based on his book *Through the Red Sea, A Path to Private Care*, in which he describes "The Journey of a Dentist dealing with the encroachment of corporate dentistry by creating a high-quality, patient-centered, fee-for-service practice." By removing himself from insurance networks and leading with a health-centered practice philosophy, Michael successfully positioned his practice as the go-to location for exceptional comprehensive care. He now teaches others how to do the same on both the technical and behavioral levels. You can learn more by contacting Michael at www.theschustercenter.com

***

Susan Maples, of Holt, Michigan practices and teaches "Total Health Dentistry," about which she says, "It turns out that your mouth has a great deal to say about the rest of your body." Susan leverages her understanding of oral health to "predict and preempt systemic diseases such as heart disease, diabetes, sleep apnea, acid reflux, chronic systemic inflammation, food sensitivities, oral cancer, chemical sensitivity, and more." Susan is a popular speaker and has written two books titled: *Brave Parent: Raising Healthy, Happy Kids Against All Odds in Today's World*, and *BlabberMouth! 77 Secrets Only Your Mouth Can Tell You*. Susan can be reached at www.totalhealth-dentistry.com

***

Alice Lam is a graduate of the University of Texas Health Sciences at San Antonio School of Dentistry. Alice practices in Houston, where she collaborates with other medical professionals to advance *Integrative Medicine,* wherein they view the body as a complex set of interrelated systems that, when out of balance, can symptomatically present in various ways. Alice is a former visiting faculty member of the Pankey Institute and has since created the *Align Center for Integrative Health and Postural Restoration,* where she helps her patients overcome dysfunctional postural adaptations, many of which symptomatically present in the head, neck, temporomandibular joint system, and airway. Alice can be contacted at www.smilesourcewesthouston.com

***

Tom Colquitt, is a private practitioner, former adjunct professor at the Baylor College of Dentistry, the LSU School of Medicine, and Past President of the American Academy of Restorative Dentistry. Tom has dedicated the last 20 years of his life to helping people overcome breathing disorders by facilitating their "walk to wellness." Functional nasodiaphragmatic breathing is Tom's treatment goal, which is achieved through habit change, positive functional adaptations, orthodontics, surgically-assisted orthodontics, and/or restorative dentistry. As Tom says, "The most important muscle in the body is the heart, and the second most important is the diaphragm." You can view Tom's presentation on how he improved his own health and the health of his patients on his YouTube video series titled *Stories from the Road.*

***

Jeff Rouse, is a prosthodontist in private practice, adjunct professor at the University of Texas, and faculty member of Spear Education™. In 2013, Jeff published *Sleep Prosthodontics: A New Vision for Dentistry,* and has become a leading voice in helping us to better understand the relationship between airway health and oral health. Jeff can be contacted at www.rousedds.com

***

Jeffrey Hoos of Stratford, Connecticut is a restorative dentist and popular speaker who developed the *Teeth for a Lifetime* periodontal evaluation and therapy program, a patient-centered, interactive clinical protocol used to evaluate and treat periodontal disease. The program includes a written *Treatment Partnership*

Plan that emphasizes the patient's role as co-therapist, similar to the Barkley model. To learn more, visit www.bettersmile.com

***

Kevin Boyd is a board-certified pediatric dentist with extensive experience delivering healthcare to infants, children, adolescents, and young adults with physical and/or mental disabilities, and other special needs. After graduating from Loyola University's Chicago College of Dentistry in 1986, he attended the University of Iowa for his advanced residency training in Pediatric Dentistry. Kevin also holds an advanced degree (M.Sc.) in Human Nutrition and Dietetics from Michigan State University, where he participated in research projects related to unhealthy eating and how it contributes to tooth decay, obesity and Type 2 Diabetes. His strong academic background in nutritional biochemistry has been instrumental in motivating the importance he places on nutrition as being a key component of each child's dental health plan. Kevin is recognized as a leading clinician in the country for diagnosing and treating interferences to normal growth of the teeth, jaws and face. He teaches an advanced mini-residency on guiding early childhood facial development in collaboration with Dr. Ben Miraglia and Airway Health Solutions. info@airwayhealthsolutions.com

***

Ben Miraglia of Mount Kisco, New York, is a general dentist focused on full mouth restorative dentistry in combination with guiding growth and development through orthodontics, with a particular emphasis on the use of Invisalign®, with which he has had a long-time faculty association. He lectures internationally on how to deploy non-extraction/non-surgical orthodontics for airway development and management. Additionally, he founded Airway Health Solutions®, an educational/consulting company that teaches dental professionals to "combat malocclusion and sleep-disordered breathing via craniofacial development, expansive/interceptive orthodontics and myofascial therapy for airway health." Ben can be contacted at info@airwayhealthsolutions.com

***

Steven Lamberg is a comprehensive restorative dentist in Northport, New York, as well as the Scientific Advisor for Airway Management at *The Kois Center.* He is a Diplomate of the American Board of Dental Sleep Medicine, and the inventor of the *Lamberg SleepWell Appliance*, designer of the *Lamberg Airway and Sleep Navigator* form, and author of *Treat the Cause…Treat the Airway:* The Role of Snoring & Sleep Apnea in Contemporary Preventive Medicine. Steven can be contacted at https://drlamberg.com

***

The Pankey Institute has long been a resource for learning more about health-centered, comprehensive dentistry that's integrated into a whole-person approach, which includes understanding patients on the physical, psychological, and learning levels. That approach is paralleled by helping dentists and team members learn how to do the same thing – to understand themselves better on the physical, psychological, and learning levels so they can become better facilitators of health. The Pankey curriculum is extensive and worth considering if you need a place to start or to continue your professional development. The Institute's curriculum can be viewed at www.pankey.org

***

In spite of these examples of exceptional leadership, the future of person-centered, health-centered dentistry is in *your* hands as the current generation of thought leaders passes the proverbial baton. By writing this book, it is my hope that I have inspired you to take action in that direction. Peter Drucker famously said, "The greatest danger in times of turbulence is not the turbulence; it's to act with yesterday's logic." Drucker's statement is an evergreen truth in dentistry; we must keep moving forward as we simultaneously leverage the wisdom and logic of Robert F. Barkley.

Afterword

The roots of this book descend into the earliest days of my professional career. I settled in Lexington, Kentucky after graduation from the University of Michigan School of Dentistry, just like my father, and uncle decades before me. Lexington was my choice because it was where I had completed my undergraduate work, and where I'd fallen in love with the central Kentucky lifestyle. I landed two assistant professorships at the College of Dentistry and an associate position in a practice on the southwest side of town.

I enjoyed teaching while I simultaneously struggled to get my "real world" experience launched due to a local ratio of one dentist per 900 residents. My associate position was a replacement role for a former partner who'd left dentistry to sell Shaklee® nutritional supplements. That was the first negative signal that went right over my head. The second signal was related to the departing partner not having enough patients to fill my schedule, and the third signal was located in the lab, where multiple case pans full of crowns and bridgework sat undelivered—many of them made several years earlier. When I asked Ron why, he nonchalantly answered, "They didn't want to pay their co-payment, so they never came back."

Ron and I got along fine, but unbeknownst to me, I was expected to grow my own practice. I was a virtual stranger in a city overflowing with dentists. Almost everyone was under contract with every form of dental insurance, including HMO, PPO, and capitation plans, which was the only way to market outside of the Yellow Pages® which had eight pages of double-truck display ads, or newspaper ads that were even more expensive.

Within a year, I decided to take a chance on a start-up office near the University. It was in a new development that had leased space to a nice restaurant, boutique shops, and had a number of upscale condominiums nearby. I rationalized to myself that with so many people living, working, and shopping nearby, my convenient location would be a perfect fit into their lives. My strategy was only partly successful, after learning how difficult it is to get people to change dentists—even when they're dissatisfied. I had to combine my income from the University, a Saturday associateship in Pikeville, and my new practice to make the math work.

Over time, I started to look for a more convenient associate position that would allow me to leave the University and generate more income. That process led me to the office of Bob Muncy, a highly regarded restorative dentist. Bob was looking for an associate, an opportunity that I'd learned about through the University. His office was immaculate, upscale, fully fee-for-service, busy, and buzzing with a happy care team and patients. In other words, it was the opposite of my experience: a slow, moth-eaten schedule in spite of "taking" every insurance known to mankind. I soon learned that Bob had trained at *The Pankey Institute* and had every case mounted on a semi-adjustable articulator. Additionally, he was doing full-mouth reconstructions or significant restoration work every week, in combination with being paid a full fee with gratitude. Bob lived in a world that I didn't know existed; it amazed me and piqued my curiosity. How could he do that when my little start-up down the road was nearly on life support every month? I found the answer in Bob's private office. There, sitting on Bob's custom-built bookcase, were books from people named Dawson, Okeson, and newsletters from people named Reed and King, as well as places called *The Pankey Institute* and CRA.

I picked up Avrom King's Nexus newsletter after Bob left the room to see patients, and I couldn't put it down. Avrom wrote about topics never discussed in dental school: macro and microeconomics, marketing, "Tiers," how people learn, strategic development, team selection, team development, leadership, computerization, discriminating personalities, Carl Rogers, and some guy named Bob Barkley.

Bob gifted me all the back copies after telling him that I was fascinated with the content. At a follow-up visit, Bob told me that I needed to meet a pedodontist/orthodontist by the name of Walter Doyle. And when I did, my paradigm was destroyed yet again. Walter was the first-ever double board-certified orthodontist-pedodontist. He mounted every case on a SAM II articulator via an Axiograph®, and was part of Rudolph Slavicek's Vienna, Austria study club. Additionally, Walter had a teaching facility in the lower level of his office, where twelve dentists would train with him ten times a year for two years. While there, students stayed with Walter at his home, an antebellum mansion located on a horse farm north of town. There, they would discuss complex cases over dinner and long into the night, often focusing their attention on dental arch expansion, making room for tongues, guiding midface development, and stimulating condylar growth in children.

My conception of what dentistry *could be* was forever changed during that time, but there was a major problem with my new understanding: I couldn't experience it, because I hadn't yet prepared myself. Consequently, I spent the next twenty years studying learning, training, and applying. The self-development process led me all over the country to learn under many masters and institutions. It also took me on a life-long journey to find out more about the mysterious Bob Barkley in service to my goal: To create a truly person-centered, health-centered practice, create a teaching center, teach hands-on, and coach.

Additional outcomes of my journey are this book and the *Bob Barkley Study Club,* created as vehicles to share knowledge and experiences. If you are interested in becoming involved in the *Bob Barkley Study Club*, you can follow the Facebook page, attend a workshop, sponsor a presentation at your study club, or initiate a coaching relationship.

For more information, please visit: codisovery.com, or email paul@paulhennydds.com

I would love to hear from you.

~Paul A. Henny, DDS

Endnotes

1. Barkley, R. Successful Preventive Dental Practices, Preventive Press, 1972, p. 7

2. Barkley, R. Successful Preventive Dental Practices, Preventive Press, 1972, p. 23

3. Pankey, L.D., Davis, W. A Philosophy of the Practice of Dentistry, Medical College Press (1987): pp. 3-51

4. Conversations with Jon Barkley about Macomb while he was growing up

5. Barkley, R., Successful Preventive Dental Practices, Prevention Press, (1972): p. 13

6. Pankey, L.D., Davis, W. A Philosophy of the Practice of Dentistry, Medical College Press (1987): p. 76

7. Eulogy at Robert F. Barkley Funeral

8. Eulogy at Robert F. Barkley Funeral

9. Barkley, R., Successful Preventive Dental Practices, Prevention Press (1972): p. 11

10. Barkley, R., Successful Preventive Dental Practices, Prevention Press (1972): p. 11

11. Barkley, R., Successful Preventive Dental Practices, Prevention Press (1972): p. 11

12. Barkley, R. Successful Preventive Dental Practices, Prevention Press, (1972): p. 13

13. Barkley, R. Successful Preventive Dental Practices, Prevention Press, (1972): pp. 18-19

14. Barkley, R. Successful Preventive Dental Practices, Prevention Press, (1972): p. 21

15. Barkley, Robert. Successful Preventive Dental Practices, Prevention Press (1972): pp. 91-99

16. Eulogy, Bob Barkley Funeral (1977)

17. Barkley, Robert. Successful Preventive Dental Practices, Prevention Press (1972): p. 28

18. Barkley, R., Lecture, Emory University Dental School (Recorded 1973)

19. Southam, Wilson. Volitional Practice, A Powerful Way of Living and Practicing, The Phoenix Academy, Tape Series (1987)

20. Southam, Wilson. Volitional Practice, A Powerful Way of Living and Practicing, The Phoenix Academy, Tape Series (1987)

21. Barkley, R., On Becoming A Humanistic Dentist, The Nexus Group (1977) p3

22. Barkley, R., Successful Preventive Dental Practices, Prevention Press (1972) p. 76

23. Barkley, R., Lecture, Emory University Dental School Presentation (1973)

24. L.D. Pankey and W.J Davis. A Philosophy of the Practice of Dentistry, Medical College Press (1987) p. 3-10

25. ORS Faculty: John Anderson, Herb Gustavson, Meig Jones, Gerard Courtade, John Wilson, Dave Hoffman, F. Harold Wirth, Gus Perdigon, and Loren Miller

26. Trial Run Class: Herbert Gustavson, Meigs Jones, Earl Poe, Dwight Hudson, Bob King, David Hildebrand, Keith Thornton, Bill Bryant, and Richard Green

27. Original Cadre: Richard Alpert, Fred Begeman, Bill Bryant,

28. Fred Cory, Roy Cowen, Donald Culp, Richard Green, Bill Griffith, Guy Haddix, David Hildebrand, Bill Lockard, Jr., Ed Quinn, Mike Schuster, Keith Thornton, Tymon Totte

29. 1973-4 Board of Directors: John A. Anderson, W. L. Butterworth, Jr., James Cosper, Jr., William Dolan, Edward Green, Herbert Gustavson, Robert C. King, Loren Miller, Frank T.Scott, F. Harold Wirth, Jack R. Wilkins.

30. 1973-4 Board of Trustees: John A. Anderson, L.W. Anderson, Jr., Robert Barkley, George Colman, James Cosper, Jr., Peter E. Dawson, William Dolan, John Flower, Herbert Gustavson, David Hoffman, S. Meigs Jones, Robert C. King, Loren Miller, Gustave Perdigon, Earl Poe, Jr., Rose H. Quick, Clyde H. Schuyler, Frank T. Scott, Glenn A. Thomas, John O. Wilson, F. Harold Wirth.

31. Barkley, R. Successful Preventive Dental Practices, Prevention Press (1972) pp. 232-233

32. Barkley, R. Successful Preventive Dental Practices, Prevention Press (1972) pp. 232-233

33. Barkley, R. Successful Preventive Dental Practices, Prevention Press (1972) pp. 232-233

34. Brown, William. A Profile of an Unsung Hero, InASpritofCaring.com (2016)

35. Barkley, R., Successful Preventive Dental Practices, Prevention Press (1972) p. 16

36. Personal communications with Paul A. Henny, DDS

37. King, Avrom. The Nitty Gritty of New Dentistry, King and Company, Cassette Tape Series (1985)

38. Personal communications with Rich Green, DDS, MBA (1999)

39. An Interview with Charles Sorenson, Journal of Clinical Orthodontics, (1970) p. 1

40. An Interview with Charles Sorenson, Journal of Clinical Orthodontics, (1970) p. 1

41. An interview with Charles Sorenson, Journal of Clinical Orthodontics (1970) p. 2

42. Personal communications with Rich Green, DDS, MBA (1999)

43. An interview with Charles Sorenson, Journal of Clinical Orthodontics (1970) p. 2

44. Personal communications with Rich Green, DDS, MBA (1999)

45. Benko, R. Forty Years Ago, Today Nixon Took Us Off the Gold Standard (2011) https//:www.foxnews.com/gold

46. PFC Capital, Private Equity Investment in Dental Care Creating Long-term Value, (2023) www.providenthp.com

47. Janse, B. (2021) Rational Goal Model. Retrieved 2/2/2023 from Toolshero: https://toolshero.com/management/rational-goal-model/p. 1

48. Brook, M. (2002) Planning Theory for Practitioners. Chicago: American Planning Association. pp. 175-176

49. Chen, P. (2013). For New Doctors, 8 Minutes Per Patient. Retrieved 2/2/2023 from archieve.nytimes.com, p. 1

50. Although the following experience isn't true for every dentist, it's indicative of the meta-trend: "I graduated in 2020, and worked for a DSO since. I would advise any new grad to try to find any option besides corporate. I can honestly say I'm already incredibly burnt out. I've had no real mentorship or clinical help since I graduated. I truly hate dentistry now. All they care about is milking production out of you with no regard for your well-being.

I understand it's hard to stay away, but trust me, if you can you should." (Anonymous Facebook post January 2023)

51. Pankey L.D., Wirth, F. H. (1986) A Philosophy of the Practice of Dentistry, Audio Recording, Denver Colorado

52. Wirth, F. H. (1985) Interview with Dr. F. Harold Wirth, The Portal to Texas History, Video Recording: Texashistory.unt.edu

53. Pankey L.D., Wirth, F. H. (1986) A Philosophy of the Practice of Dentistry, Audio Recording, Denver Colorado

54. Pankey L.D., Wirth, F. H. (1986) A Philosophy of the Practice of Dentistry, Audio Recording, Denver Colorado

55. Pankey L.D., Wirth, F. H. (1986) A Philosophy of the Practice of Dentistry, Audio Recording, Denver Colorado

56. Pankey L.D., Wirth, F. H. (1986) A Philosophy of the Practice of Dentistry, Audio Recording, Denver Colorado

57. Robichaux, M., Keynote Address F. Harold Wirth Foundation, LSU School of Dentistry (2014)

58. Research for this chapter was conducted by interviewing Richard A. Green and email communications for confirmation.

59. Barkley, R. Successful Preventive Dental Practices, Prevention Press (1972) p.76

60. Baker, D. Reflections on Rogers. PSYCH TODAY, (2012) https://www.psychologicalscience.org/observer/reflections-on-rogers.

61. Cherry, K (2023). Humanistic Psychology: Definition and History. Accessed 2/2/2023 https://www.explorepsychology.com

62. Rogers, C., Client-Centered Therapy. Boston: Houghton-Mifflin; (1951): pp 7-130

63. Rogers, C., Client-Centered Therapy. Boston: Houghton-Mifflin; (1951): pp 7-130

64. Source: multiple conversations with Mike Schuster

65. Schuster, M., Practice-building with the Dental Fitness Program, The Center for Professional Development (1985)

66. King, A., The Nitty Gritty of New Dentistry, audio tape series (1982)

67. Research for this chapter was conducted through a personal interview with Mary Osbourne.

68. Barkley, R. Successful Preventive Dental Practices, Prevention Press (1972) p.72

69. Research of this chapter was conducted via interviews and confirmation emails.

70. An excellent tribute to Omer Reed's writing, thinking, and presentations was lovingly created by John Highsmith and is available to explore at www.omerreed.com

71. Research for this chapter was based upon personal correspondence and an interview with William Strupp, Jr.

72. Maltz, M., Psycho-Cybernetics, Tarcher-Perigree (1960)

73. Heidegger, Martin, Biographical Sketch, Accessed 2/2/2023 plato.stanford.edu (2011)

74. Barkley, R. Successful Preventive Dental Practices, Prevention Press (1972) p.15

75. Carlisle, L. (1994). In a Spirit of Caring, Kendall/Hunt (1994) pp.37-41

76. Carlisle, L. (1994). In a Spirit of Caring, Kendall/Hunt (1994) pp.37-41

77. 2 Frazer, R. (2014) Bob Frazer Writes About Bob Barkley, Accessed 1/4/2018 inaspiritofcaring.com

78. Jung Society of Washington, Accessed 2/2/2023 http://jung.org

79. King, A., Choosing to Choose, Praxis Press (1998) pp.85-93

80. Research for this chapter was conducted via interview and validation for accuracy by email with Gary DeWood.

81. Beattie, M., Codependent No More, How to Stop Controlling Others and Start Caring for Yourself, Spiegel & Grau (2022) 7-18

82. McGregor, D., The Human Side of Enterprise. McGraw Hill (1960) pp 17-23

83. Esfahani-Smith, E., The Power of Meaning, Finding Fulfillment in a World Obsessed with Happiness, (2017) Crown Publishing, pp 46-49

84. Achor, S., The Happiness Advantage:How a Positive Brain Fuels Success in Work and Life, (2018) Currency pub.

85. Baumeister, Vohs, et al. (2013) Some Key Differences Between a Happy Life and A Meaningful Life. Journal of Positive Psychology, Vol. 8, Issue 6, pp 505-516

86. King, A., Managing for Excellence, The Nexus Group, (1987) audio cassette series

87. Research of this chapter was conducted via interview and verification via confirmation emails with Brian Vence.

88. Panksepp, Y. (2012) The Archeology of the Mind,

89. Neuroevolutionary Origins of Human Emotions, W.W. Norton

90. Bradshaw, J. (2005) Healing the Shame that Binds You, Health Communications Inc; Revised edition

91. Barkley, R., Lecture, Emory University Dental School, (Recorded 1973)

92. Research for this chapter was conducted by an interview, and then the content was confirmed by email with M.J. Hagood.

93. Dr. Steve Hart added: "Johnson Hagood is the kid-brother I never had. I have known him since before he started dental school, and watching him find his way in this profession we both love has been a joy beyond words. He has been on that "Hero's journey," and he certainly is one of my heroes! I could not be prouder of my kid-brother!"

94. Sorensen, C., An Interview with Charles Sorensen, Journal of Clinical Orthodontics (1980)

95. Leung, J., Grant, M. (2022) Jean Piaget's Disequilibrium &

96. Accommodation Theory, Accessed 2/2/2023 http://www.study.com

97. Huseman-Kopetzky, M. (2018) Handbook on the Psychology of Pricing, Pricing School Press

98. Barkley, R. Successful Preventive Dental Practices, Prevention Press (1972) p.182

99. Siegel, D., The Mindful Therapist, A Clinician's Guide to

100. Mindsight and Neural Integration, W.W.Norton & Co. (2010) pp 56-57

101. Tooth Decay, National Institute of Dental Craniofacial Research (April 2019) NIH Accessed 2/2/2023 www.ada.org/resources/research/science-and-research-institute/oral-health-topics/periodontitis

102. Slowik, JM, et al, Obstructive Sleep Apnea. StatPearls Publishing LLC. (2022) Accessed 2/2/2023 www.ncbi.nlm.nih.gov

103. Egnew, TR, Suffering, Meaning, and Healing: Challenges of Contemporary Medicine, The Annals of Family Medicine (March 2009) 7 (2) 170-175

104. Barkley, R., Lecture, Emory University Dental School Presentation, (Recorded 1973)

105. Evaluation of a Daily Oral Care Lozenge on Oral Health and Quality of Life in Older Adults, Clinical Trials.gov; U.S. National Library of Medicine (Oct. 2018)